Breast Health Handbook

Breast Health Handbook

Compiled by Caryn Franklin and Georgina Goodman
in association with BREAKTHROUGH Breast Cancer

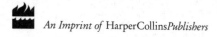

An Imprint of HarperCollins*Publishers*

Pandora
An Imprint of HarperCollins*Publishers*
77–85 Fulham Palace Road,
Hammersmith, London W6 8JB
1160 Battery Street,
San Francisco, California 94111–1213

Published by Pandora 1996

10 9 8 7 6 5 4 3 2 1

© compilation BREAKTHROUGH Breast Cancer 1996

© each contribution remains with individual authors

BREAKTHROUGH Breast Cancer and the contributors to
this book assert the moral right to be identified
as the authors of this work

A catalogue record for this book
is available from the British Library

ISBN 0 04 440979 6

Printed in Great Britain by
Woolnough Bookbinding Limited, Irthlingborough, Northamptonshire

Contents

Part III: The Whole Body: The Whole Picture

Part IV: If You Find a Lump

Part V: Surgery

Part VI: Fighting Back

Part VII: Feelings

Part VIII: Science and Research: Now and the Future

Part IX: Useful Information

A Note from
BREAKTHROUGH Breast Cancer

Dear Reader

Thank you for buying this book, which marks the launch of Fashion Targets Breast Cancer – a major campaign backed by the British fashion industry to raise funds for BREAKTHROUGH Breast Cancer. With this purchase you have already made a contribution towards helping BREAKTHROUGH establish Britain's first dedicated Breast Cancer Research Centre.

Breast cancer kills 15,000 women every year – that's one woman almost every half hour – and it is on the increase. BREAKTHROUGH wants to change all this by bringing together top scientists and doctors under one roof in a co-ordinated campaign of research focused exclusively on this one disease. By creating such a centre of excellence, we believe that we will create the best possible environment for finding a cure. BREAKTHROUGH's Centre will be a joint development with the Institute of Cancer Research, and will be situated on London's Fulham Road, alongside the Royal Marsden Hospital. The progress made by the scientists who will work within it will benefit every single woman in this country, and all over the world.

BREAKTHROUGH's new Centre is due to open in 1998 but, even before it is up and running, BREAKTHROUGH has begun to fund two crucial research projects, worth a total of £1.6 million. Already the charity has played a vital role in the recent discovery of the second breast cancer gene, BRCA2, which will ultimately enable early diagnosis of women who may be at risk of developing the disease.

Fashion Targets Breast Cancer is BREAKTHROUGH's major fundraising campaign for 1996. One in 12 women develops breast cancer at some stage in her life. If one in 12 of you buys a Fashion Targets Breast Cancer T-shirt as well as this book, we will raise more than £20 million towards our goal.

Thank you so much for your support.

Delyth Morgan
Chief Executive, BREAKTHROUGH Breast Cancer
London, February 1996

If you would like to find out more about BREAKTHROUGH's campaign, or make a donation, please call 0171–405 5111 or write to BREAKTHROUGH Breast Cancer, PO Box LB25, London WC2B 6QW.

Foreword

DR DIANA TAIT

Most women are aware of breast cancer, either as a risk to themselves or as a disease that has affected family, friends or colleagues; media interest in the subject has also raised its profile. However, the information available through the media tends to be fragmented, incomplete, indigestible or even inaccurate. As a result, it can induce panic rather than leading to better understanding.

This handbook provides a comprehensive exploration of the subject of breast health, breast awareness and breast cancer, and presents it in a way that is accessible. In fact it makes rather compelling reading. Unlike the impenetrable nature of many sources of information, here is a superb mix of the scientific, technical, philosophical and personal; the clear explanation of scientific issues is balanced by the enormously valuable inclusion of practical advice, making the whole subject much more accessible. A particularly useful section is the Directory, which includes relevant contact addresses and telephone numbers.

I think this book will be of enormous benefit to all women, and it needn't be read exhaustively as each of the sections is complete and will allow readers to dip in and out according to their interests. It is the sort of book that all women should have on their shelves; those who are having to deal with breast cancer at closer quarters will find in it a clear, calm and empathetic approach.

Dr Diana Tait
Royal Marsden Hospital NHS Trust
London, February 1996

Preface

RALPH LAUREN

When my very dear friend Nina Hyde, a former *Washington Post* fashion editor, died of breast cancer in 1991 I was confronted with the pain that this disease can cause. Nina, whose faith remained steadfast despite very real obstacles, was my guiding force in the fight against breast cancer. While Nina may have lost her personal battle, I know she'd be so proud of how Fashion Targets Breast Cancer has proved that, by banding together, we can and do make a difference.

In the United States we have raised US$2 million, with the support of so many people across the country, and we have also raised awareness of one of the most dreadful diseases of our time. In the US one in nine women will develop breast cancer at some time in her life. This is a truly frightening statistic, but I believe we have it in our power to change it. We will educate, raise funds and do everything it takes until breast cancer is completely abolished.

The concern of the fashion industry about breast cancer is a global one. Fashion Targets Breast Cancer has already raised another US$2 million for breast cancer research in Brazil. Now that Britain has taken up this important cause, I hope this will be the beginning of a series of European campaigns. I am so pleased and proud to have been able to begin an initiative that has caught the imagination and commitment of so many in our industry from many parts of the world.

I wish you all the greatest success with your British campaign. Thank you for your support.

Ralph Lauren
New York, February 1996

Acknowledgements

We would like to thank all those who have contributed their time and expertise to this book; most especially the writers who have striven to meet such tight deadlines. Thanks to Professor Barry Gusterson of the Institute of Cancer Research, who has been on the end of the phone throughout, helping with the smallest enquiry to the biggest problem. It goes without saying that we couldn't have done it without you. Your time and commitment have been invaluable. And to Sally Townsend, Professor Gusterson's secretary, for her calm handling of our frenzied calls. Our thanks to Anna Maslin, who has given considerable advice and support. Many students have given their time to help with this book – Abigail Rayner, Juliet Yashar, Donna Richmond, Olivia Auger and Liz Reid – thank you all. Special thanks to Lindsey Fay from Central St Martin's; Lee Widows, course director at Central St Martin's, for motivating her journalism students; and Josie Kemp, course director at the Surrey Institute of Art and Design, whose students attacked this project with gusto. Thank you also to Colette Foster and Roger Casstles of the BBC's *The Clothes Show*, who have given valuable support to this project and have been instrumental in the progress of Fashion Targets Breast Cancer.

A BIG 'thank you' to Belinda Budge at Pandora and all her team for believing in this book and getting right behind it, and our very appreciative thanks to Sara Dunn at Pandora, who had the challenge of turning the organic matter into a literate organ.

Thank you to Val Holmes from the Guild of Health Writers for her interest and support. A 'we couldn't have done it without you!'-style thank you to Suzanne Marston, who typed round the clock to meet our deadline; and also 'thank you Dad' to Caryn's father, who breathed life back into our tired old printer at the eleventh hour.

Thank you B. J. Cunningham, Ian Denyer, Mateda Franklin Saldaan and Emma Dunk for your constant love and support on the home front.

Finally, a heartfelt thank you to Lyn Brown and all the women from the BREAKTHROUGH Breast Cancer regional networks, especially the women who have generously shared their lives in this book. From you we have learnt a great deal.

Introduction: Fashion Targets Breast Cancer

I heard about the campaign Fashion Targets Breast Cancer in 1995 when I attended a meeting in the Holborn offices of the charity BREAKTHROUGH Breast Cancer. Ralph Lauren was instrumental in launching the US campaign following the death of his close friend and colleague Nina Hyde, former fashion editor of the *Washington Post*. His efforts united the entire American fashion industry in pursuit of fund- and awareness-raising on the subject of breast cancer.

Spurred into action by the importance of such a campaign, the Council of Fashion Designers of America, including household names such as Calvin Klein, Donna Karan and Oscar de la Renta as well as hot new names like Anna Sui, Todd Oldham and Isaac Mizrahi, supported this bold and powerful initiative by capturing the attention of the American public. Over 350,000 Fashion Targets Breast Cancer T-shirts were sold in stores across North America, and US$2 million raised. As well as founding the Nina Hyde Centre, the American fashion industry established breast cancer as a major topic of debate, generating an unprecedented wave of press interest and, perhaps just as importantly, creating an extremely successful money-raising formula for other countries to follow.

Two years on, as we sat in BREAKTHROUGH Breast Cancer's offices and were shown the phenomenal press coverage, T-shirts, promotional videos and ads of the US campaign, I was asked, along with other representatives from the British fashion industry, if it would be possible to organize a similar campaign in Britain.

I was instantly attracted to the idea, for many reasons. Our own Jean Muir had died of breast cancer some months before, and I also knew of others within the industry who were battling against the illness. In my time as a fashion journalist and television presenter I have witnessed the courage many women show in the face of this particularly cruel cancer. In the Breast Cancer Care Road Shows, all the models who parade the catwalk have recovered from breast surgery. Gracing the walkway like veteran nymphets in their plunging necklines and saucy swimsuits, these women may often still be negotiating worries about their own health and future. I have much admiration for the way in which personal anxieties are confronted in order to offer reassurance to every woman in the audience. For inspiration and beauty, these catwalk shows beat the offerings of a top Parisian couturier any day.

But there were other grounds for my interest. The fashion industry is rightly perceived by many as a superficial business, concerned only with trivia and visual gloss. Women's bodies, central to the very existence of fashion designers and their creative urges, are frequently treated like alabaster deities there to be adored and adorned. The subtext of course is that only those with immaculately formed frames, those whose mathematically perfect bodies conform to the rigid definitions of western beauty (strenuously policed by the fashion industry itself), are invited to enjoy this lavish attention. In actively campaigning on behalf of a breast cancer research charity, here was a chance for the fashion world to declare loyalty to the bodies of all women – and more importantly to offer a service dedicated to fundamental issues of health and life. This is a campaign for mothers, daughters, partners, wives, grandmothers, sisters, aunts and friends. It is for those who care about issues other than hemlines or news from the frontline of Paris or Milan. The statistics for breast-cancer-related deaths are alarming; the equivalent, in fact, to a jumbo jet full of women passengers crashing every fortnight. A breast cancer diagnosis also leaves many more to deal with life without one or both breasts, with various other health complications, and a future of uncertainties.

In the days after that first meeting I considered the responsibility. I explored my own ignorance, and shared this lack of knowledge with others. I realized (despite the deluge of magazine articles) that I was ill-informed, and so were many of my contemporaries. Some years ago I discovered a lump while lying in bed; it had immediately caused me a lot of panic. But a visit to the clinic and an examination using ultra-sound imagery accompanied by a maternal squeeze of the hand from the nurse reassured me enough to return to my life without another thought. I hadn't bothered to learn much about breast cancer along the way. Later, one of my sisters had several lumps removed from both breasts. She didn't explain much of what had happened – or maybe I didn't ask. As I considered the experiences of various friends and acquaintances, my desire to take on this campaign grew.

I began to sound out my colleagues, and almost instantly senior people on *The Clothes Show* consented to advance the cause. *The Clothes Show* decided to schedule an item on Fashion Targets Breast Cancer, guaranteed to reach millions of women up and down the country. They also agreed to donate considerable resources for the making of a promotional video to be shown in shopping malls and individual retail outlets across the land. Meanwhile, award-winning evening wear designer Amanda Wakeley, who is chair of the campaign, enlisted the enthusiasm and editorial brawn of Alex Shulman, editor of British *Vogue*. With a headquarters now established in the heart of Condé Nast Publishing, a meeting was set for designers and retailers to discuss the selling of T-shirts. The fashion world had begun to target breast cancer.

I travelled to Milan and, in the course of making our usual collection report for the programme, I interviewed well-known names for the campaign. Supermodel Helena Christensen was the first to declare her interest, refusing all other interview requests backstage at Gianfranco Ferre. She spoke about the subject with knowledge and passion, as did many of the world's most beautiful women I questioned that day. Since then I have pointed a microphone in the direction of numerous members of the British fashion fraternity, including Bruce Oldfield, Betty Jackson, Nicole Farhi, Vidal Sassoon, Marie Helvin, Kate Moss, Roland Klein, Caroline Charles, John Galliano, Ally Capellino and Zandra Rhodes, all of whom spoke eloquently and were keen to enlist.

At a meeting later in London, representatives from the UK's most powerful retailing giants added their corporate might, consenting to sell the T-shirts in their stores and shops up and down the country, unanimously refusing the traditional mark-up to encourage more sales and to ensure that every penny spent by members of the public went straight to BREAK-THROUGH Breast Cancer. M. & C. Saatchi accepted the assignment of promoting the entire event using a billboard campaign, tube posters and magazine adverts, while Gianni Versace's British PR, Aurelia Public Relations, took on the immense task of co-ordinating all the elements of this now huge concern and translating it into material that newspaper, magazine and television journalists could use.

From the beginning I had suggested a campaign book. Not one that was frivolous and self-congratulatory, but a solid awareness-raising tool, to perform the twin functions of raising money and consciousness, and dispensing practical information, advice and contacts. But the challenge of making it happen in such a short time seemed enormous. My working partner Georgina Goodman and I began to track down some of the country's most prestigious health and medical experts. Telephones trilled in offices up and down the country, faxes snaked out statistics, and we feverishly tried to make contact. One by one, well-known writers and health experts like Liz Earle, Dr Miriam Stoppard, Susan Curtis (founder of Neal's Yard Remedies), Anne Hooper (psycho/sexual counsellor) and Vivienne Parry (*Tomorrow's World* scientist) agreed to donate their writing and ideas. Respected journalists from a wide range of popular newspapers and women's magazines joined our masthead, as well as medical specialists recommended by Professor Barry Gusterson at the Institute of Cancer Research. The book began to take shape in a matter of days.

Pandora, well-known for their attention to women's health, expressed an interest in the idea. At this point it seemed an impossibility for any large publishing company to meet the tight deadlines we had. But they did, and the fact that this book happened at all owes as much to the determination of many women and men in the book trade as it does to the breast cancer specialists.

Epidemiology, oncology ... you name it, we've looked it up. And here we speak the truth, because our knowledge of this subject was scant to non-existent. But within such ignorance lies the key to the book you now have in your hand. We may have compiled it, but we are also its readers. The information contained within this handbook has been carefully planned to begin at the beginning and explain fully the subjects of breast health, breast awareness and breast disease. It takes in the knowledge of a range of experts in varied fields and tries to combine readability with expertise. Other experts, such as the women who have generously shared their own experience of breast cancer, beam a light on a path already trodden by them but unfamiliar to others. There is a Glossary at the back of the book to help with terminology (which can sometimes seem intimidating), and a Directory of contacts, supplied by the contributing writers, to ensure that you can follow up suggestions for help. Finally there's a Further Reading list for those of you who, like me, want to research particular areas of interest. The belief we all have in producing this book is that information is a vital component in understanding how to take responsibility for our health.

Fashion Targets Breast Cancer is a campaign of great importance. For too long activists, campaigners and doctors have petitioned alone for more information, more money for research and more resources for those women affected. Their voices have often been ignored, refuted or dismissed. Now the fashion industry, with its bright lights and extravagant cast, would like to add its collective voice to the demands being made. This is a time for us all to fight for improved conditions, knowledge and resources, not just for women struggling with breast cancer today but for our daughters and our grand-daughters tomorrow.

The fashion industry can help make a difference. And we all take that very seriously indeed.

Caryn Franklin
London, February 1996

Breasts Explained

The sad loss of Nina Hyde, who was a wonderful fashion journalist and supported me from the beginning of my career, made me aware of the reality of this terrible disease. I wholeheartedly support Fashion Targets Breast Cancer.
Vivienne Westwood

As we all know, breast cancer is a devastating disease. I want to help in any way I can, and I give my wholehearted support to the Fashion Targets Breast Cancer campaign.
John Rocha

1

The breast: what it's made of and what it's for

DEBORAH HUTTON

To poets, artists, lovers and every suckling infant, the breast is unique amongst human organs. Celebrated through history for its beauty and infinite variety, the truth is that scientists who spend their time looking down microscopes find this glorious orb anatomically rather ordinary, having much in common – and indeed being virtually indistinguishable from – many more mundane parts of the body.

Embryologists put us in the picture. Just six weeks after fertilization the growing embryo develops little pockets in its skin, which are destined to become the sweat glands, salivary glands and mammary glands of the fully developed individual. In later life these glands have many physiological similarities. They are composed very largely of fat; they contain an intricate interconnecting network of ducts and buds; they secrete substances (which in the case of the breast is of course milk); and, should malignancy occur in any of these organs, pathologists will tell you that the resulting tumours display strikingly similar characteristics.

Not only are all mammals alike in having mammary glands with which they feed their young, but humans can even be shown to have a vestigial 'milk line' similar to the dual rows of teats on the whelping she-dog.

Very occasionally the line can be traced by the appearance of a supernumerary third or fourth nipple, usually no more odd looking than a skin blemish or wart. These extra 'breasts' have been known to swell, and even to produce sufficient milk to feed an infant. This phenomenon, known as 'witches' milk', was one of the signs that led to certain women being branded and burned as witches in the Middle Ages.

The breasts of boys and girls are indistinguishable in childhood, containing a few rudimentary milk ducts and a little fat. During the first week or two after birth the breast tissue may swell slightly in infants of either sex. The tiny nipples may even secrete a milk-like fluid.

It is only at puberty that girls' breasts begin to take shape. In the eleventh, twelfth or thirteenth year, as the girl reaches a key 'set' weight, generally around 40 kg, a chain of events is set in motion and puberty begins. The pituitary gland at the base of the brain stimulates the production of follicles in the ovary, which in turn produces the important hormones oestrogen and progesterone. (Although oestrogen is usually referred to in the singular, there are several different types, all with subtly different functions.) The result of this inner endocrine upheaval is plainly visible in the changing contours of the female torso: the breasts enlarge, the hips widen and the pubic hair begins to sprout. Under the influence of oestrogen, the areola (darker area around the nipple) increases in size, along with the nipple itself, and the breast starts to swell as more fat is laid down and the intricate branching system of ducts and lobules starts to bud and develop.

So much is standard. What is not standard is the huge variation in shape, size and orientation of the fully-developed female breast. According to surveys, few women are satisfied with their own breast shape and size, however well endowed. Culturally, of course, very different sizes and shapes of breasts come in for veneration. The Padung tribe, for example, likes them long and pendulous, while the Maoris prefer them full and generous. Our own western ideal, which the writer Naomi Wolf has dubbed 'the official breast', is rather more compact.

In all the fuss about breasts as sexual symbols, one key point is often overlooked: the breast and of course the nipple, with its myriad nerve-endings and rich blood supply, is a huge source of sexual pleasure for billions of women, as well as billions of men, the world over. Forget Freud's distinctions between clitoral and vaginal orgasms – Kinsey, and Masters and Johnson, found a significant number of the women in their research samples could climax on stimulation of the breasts alone.

So what is the breast made of? Well, fat may be a feminist issue, but it is also a feminine tissue. Fully four-fifths of the adult female breast is fat, the rest being glandular tissue which takes the form of a branching network of tiny lobules. These connect to small ducts and from there flow into the fifteen to twenty major channels which lead directly to the nipple. A second much tinier network of tubes, this time leading centrifugally away from the nipple, contains the tissue fluid known as lymph, which accumulates in the spaces between the cells. The lymph drains through a series of thin-walled vessels into the lymph glands, which are situated both in the armpit and deep in the intercostal spaces between the ribs. The lymph glands, which are about the size and shape of kidney beans, can provide important clues as to the relative aggressiveness of breast cancer when removed for evaluation at surgery.

Contrary to popular belief, there is virtually no muscle in the breast, although there is a layer of specialized muscle-like cells in the lining of the ducts, which squeeze the milk along. The popular notion that rigorous pressing exercises can do wonders for floppy breasts is simply untrue; the breast has no muscular tissue worth writing home about. True, the pectoralis major muscle, which is responsible for the movement of the arms (among much

5

else), lies immediately under the breast. But over-exercised pects are much more likely to result in unsightly bulges under the armpit than pert bouncy bosoms. Forget pressing exercises. The best protection against droop is a well-fitting bra which will prevent gravity doing its damnedest by supporting the ligaments that hold the breast against the chest. Ligaments do not have the elastic properties of muscle: once stretched they do not spring back to shape.

As many women will know, breasts are forever changing their size, shape, consistency and sensitivity throughout the menstrual cycle, as they respond to the ebb and flow of the major ovarian hormones, oestrogen and progesterone. One recent survey of working women found that 66 per cent were aware of some degree of change in their breasts over the course of the menstrual cycle and particularly in the week before their period. Changes ranged from sensations of fullness, heaviness and tenderness to lumpiness and out-and-out pain.

Some women are more sensitive to these hormonal changes than others. Under the influence of oestrogen in the first half of the menstrual cycle, the cells lining the ducts proliferate, becoming much more plentiful and active as the breast prepares to make milk. During this time the breasts may become painfully lumpy and congested, and specific lumps may form. This is all entirely normal, and is the reason why breast experts now counsel women to be 'breast aware'. Becoming breast aware means being aware of the changes that normally happen through the phases of the menstrual cycle and, therefore, being able to recognize anything that does not feel, or look, familiar.

Many of the changes that take place in the breast in the first half of the menstrual cycle can actually be looked on as a mini-rehearsal for breast-feeding. Sometimes a tiny amount of fluid may even be released. Though this is usually instantly reabsorbed by the body, it may occasionally get trapped if there is a local overproduction of fluid or if a duct gets blocked, so that in time a cyst can form. In some cases, the cyst may become so large that a worrying lump is felt which will need aspirating (siphoning off with a long needle). Thus the lump instantaneously disappears, to the great satisfaction of both patient and doctor. Another consequence of stagnated milk secretions are the development of tiny calcium flecks, known as calcifications, which show up on a breast X-ray or mammogram. These calcifications in cysts are totally harmless. Calcifications can also be seen in association with the very early development of breast cancer, and one of the signs that the UK Breast Cancer Screening Program specifically asks radiologists to look out for when interpreting mammograms.

Most of the changes that occur in the breast are both cyclical and temporary, matching the waxing and waning of the ovarian hormones. If conception does not take place, then the changes set in motion during the first half of the menstrual cycle are not reversed. Rather they continue apace. Under the influence of steadily rising levels of oestrogen, the ducts and lobules proliferate enormously in size and number. Fat tissue increases, blood flow becomes richer and the areola surrounding the nipple becomes larger and darker, never quite returning to its original rosy pink hue. In addition, tiny clusters or buds (called acini) start to develop at the end of the lobules, which is where the milk is made. Composed of 88 per cent water, 7 per cent sugar, 4 per cent fat and 1 per cent protein, the flow of this vitamin- and antibody-rich fluid is initiated by sucking; this stimulates nerves in the nipple to release key pituitary hormones, such as prolactin, which prompts production of the milk, and oxytocin, which helps to get it flowing.

Although this all sounds very complicated, pregnancy and breastfeeding actually represent a merciful interlude of peace and quiet for the female breast compared to the hectic on-off stimulation of the menstrual cycle. The difference between the western way of life, with few children and early onset of menstruation, and the Third World lifestyle, whereby menstruation begins late and there are frequent pregnancies, is thought to have great relevance to the incidence of breast cancer, which is much more common in western society. Consider this: a woman in Britain beginning menstruation at 12, as is now the norm, may have more than four hundred menstrual cycles in her life, whereas a woman in South America, for instance, whose menstruation is delayed to the age of 16 or 17 through poverty, may have less than thirty cycles in her lifetime, as a consequence of repeated pregnancy and pro-longed breastfeeding. There is now good epidemiological evidence that the western pattern of repeated sequential hormonal stimulation of the breast by the ovaries is not good news for the breast.

Presently, some of the most forward-looking preventative efforts in this country and the US are focusing on finding a contraceptive pill that recreates the hormonal environment of the woman whose reproductive life is largely spent either pregnant or full-time breastfeeding (in which case the ovaries are effectively switched off and there is neither ovulation nor menstruation). The drug tamoxifen is very effective at preventing a second breast cancer in women who have already had one malignancy, and it is known to exert its effects in part by counteracting the effects of oestrogen (see page 66).

After all the excitement and activity of early and mid-adulthood, the breast finally quietens down at the menopause, when falling levels of oestrogen and progesterone cause the ducts within the breasts to shrink and eventually to atrophy. The breast loses volume, and the ratio of fat to glandular tissue rises yet higher, with the result that it affords a much clearer view on X-ray. One of the reasons mammography has proved so much more success-ful at picking up small cancers in women over 50 than under this age, is that there is much less going on to confuse the doctor's eye.

Although more cases of breast cancer are almost certainly associated with long-term use (more than ten years) of hormone replacement therapy, records suggest that the prospects of survival are actually *better* for such women, with the result that the mortality (death) rate from breast cancer appears no higher. As with so much in breast cancer research, the experts are still arguing fiercely about how significant this is. And they will almost certainly continue to do so well into the next century...

Thanks to Dr Peter Trott for help with this chapter.

2

Breast awareness and breast support

ANNA-MARIE SOLOWIJ

The bust business is booming. Although women have always worried about their breasts, the current focus on the breast line has prompted many to invest in the plethora of bust-enhancing treatments and underwear that has flooded the market. And women are still considering and undergoing breast augmentation, spurred on by images of well-endowed role models, many of whom have had implants. But not everyone goes under the knife for vanity's sake. Contrary to popular belief, the majority of breast augmentations are performed to correct asymmetry, where one breast is noticeably smaller than the other, or after a mastectomy or other type of breast surgery.

Breast care

Cleansing the skin of the breasts should be undertaken with care. If your breasts are large, take care to dry the folds underneath carefully, as skin rashes may occur here. Avoid using any product which could irritate the skin of the breasts. Only use preparations which are formulated for facial use. To remove hair around the nipples, use tweezers, or for permanent hair removal, visit a professional electrologist.

If you have inverted nipples, clean the nipple cavity using cotton wool buds to prevent normal secretions collecting there. Do not squeeze the nipples, as this encourages these secretions. Changes in nipple direction may occur for no known reason, but any change should be reported to your doctor. Unusual retraction – or pulling in – of the nipple may need further investigation.

Spots which occur on the breast should not be squeezed, especially if they are near the nipple, as this can lead to infection or formation of a breast abscess. When sunbathing, always take care to protect the skin of the breasts by using a cream containing a sunscreen.

Breast support

A well-fitting bra is essential for good support, and cup size is important. In order to be fitted properly with the right bra, visit your local large department store and ask to be measured, or ask for advice on how to measure yourself correctly. However, measurements only give a rough guide to size, and so you should try on a bra to make sure it fits well. You may find that your breast size changes, and different makes and styles will vary. Cup sizes range from AA (small) to DD (large), with some specialist manufacturers catering for larger sizes up to a GG fitting.

A bra should be worn as soon as the breasts start to form, even if they are small. The breasts contain fat and glandular tissue but no muscle, so it is important to prevent the ligaments, which provide natural support, from over-stretching. Good support can help to prevent drooping of the breasts, especially if they are large.

It is common to have one breast larger than the other. When choosing a bra, the bigger breast should always be used to confirm a comfortable, correct fitting. If there is a considerable difference in size it may be possible to alter the bra on the smaller side, or add some padding. Stretch bras may be useful in this situation. With underwired bras it is doubly important to ensure a correct fit so that the wires do not dig into the breast. These bras are not suitable for pregnant women or those who have had a mastectomy within the past five years.

When trying on a new bra, practise some normal stretching movements to make sure that it does not ride up and become uncomfortable.

Breast awareness

Controversy about breast self-examination remains. In favour of breast self-examination is the view that women both notice and report changes in their breasts earlier. Prompt treatment, with a wide range of available alternatives, may reduce the physical and emotional impact of breast cancer. Those who argue against breast self-examination point out that it does not prevent breast cancer or alter the course of the disease; it is therefore of little value, and can be a source of anxiety in itself. However, for some women breast self-examination has become a natural part of their lives, and there is no reason for them to change their routine.

Looking at and feeling your breasts is one way of becoming familiar with them and the usual changes that occur. In addition to general awareness you will become used to how your breasts feel throughout the month and be able to detect any differences in appearance or texture. Nine out of ten breast lumps are benign, that is, they are not cancerous. If you are unsure about what is normal for you, you could see the practice nurse at your local surgery for help and advice.

Breast awareness is more than just checking for a lump. It involves two basic steps: looking and feeling.

When looking for any changes, it helps to stand in front of a mirror. By leaning forward and moving your arms, over your head for example, you will be able to see if there are any changes in how your breasts move or in the texture of the skin, such as dimpling or puckering. Also look for any changes in the nipples, such as a change in direction, or pulling in of the nipple.

A good time to feel your breasts is in the bath or shower, using the flat of your hand when it is soapy from washing. Begin with the upper, outer part and cover the whole breast. Don't forget to feel the nipple area by pushing downwards using one finger. Squeeze the nipple gently to check for any discharge.

If you notice any of the following, consult your doctor:

- the appearance of a lump in your breast or axilla (armpit), or any area of thickening
- any dimpling or puckering of the skin on the breast
- any alteration in the appearance of the nipple or of the breast
- any discharge from the nipple.

Pain or discomfort in the breast may also indicate a condition which requires attention, for example an inflammation. If you notice any change which is unusual for you, consult your doctor; he or she will examine your breasts and may ask you to undergo some other investigations.

If you are pregnant your breasts will be undergoing changes which may be similar to some of those listed, but which are entirely normal. Ask your doctor or midwife to examine your breasts if you are concerned at all.

Benign breast disease

About one in five women will develop a form of benign breast disease at some time in her life. It is, therefore, twice as common as breast cancer, where the incidence is about one in twelve. The causes of benign breast disease are not known, but it is thought sometimes to result from an imbalance of the female sex hormones oestrogen and progesterone. Benign conditions do not appear before the onset of menstruation, when the production of these hormones begins, and are rarely seen after menopause, when production ceases.

Various conditions may occur, ranging from pain or tenderness of the breast, or nipple discharge, to a definite lump or thickening in the breasts. The symptoms frequently fluctuate in response to changes of hormone levels, especially those associated with menstruation or use of the contraceptive pill. If you experience any changes in the breast which are unusual, you should consult your doctor. He or she may ask you to return after your period to see if there is any difference in your symptoms.

Much of the information for this piece was taken from the *Patient Information Series* (No. 4) by Val Speechley published by the Royal Marsden NHS Trust.

II

Breast Cancer: An Overview

When I heard the devastating statistics that one in twelve women suffers from breast cancer and that breast cancer kills more women in Britain than any other cancer, I was determined to help in the best way I could.

The Fashion Targets Breast Cancer campaign has brought the whole fashion industry together in support of a very important cause. Our aims are to help raise awareness of breast cancer and also encourage as many people as possible to buy T-shirts in order to raise money and thereby get closer to fighting this terrible disease.

Amanda Wakeley, Chairwoman of the UK Campaign

3

Common questions about breast cancer

RITA CARTER

At what age does breast cancer usually strike?

The likelihood increases as you get older. Very few women get breast cancer in their teens and early twenties. There is no single accepted set of figures, but the chances of the average woman developing the disease before the age of 25 is about one in 20,000. The risk increases sharply with age, and experts say it roughly doubles every decade. Breast cancer is the biggest killer of women aged 40 to 50 – the mortality rate is three times that of coronary heart disease. The highest number of cases is diagnosed in the 60 to 70 age group. By the age of 85, a woman's chances of developing the disease are probably about one in ten.

Breast cancer does occur in the male breast at one per cent of the rate of occurrence in women. One of the recently discovered breast-cancer genes, BRCA2, increases the risk of both male and female breast cancer.

Does taking the pill increase one's chances of getting breast cancer?

It is still too early for definite answers – 85 per cent of women now aged under 35 have taken the pill, but the long-term effects have yet to show. Most doctors agree that any risk is almost certainly slight. The current consensus is that there is very little, or no, increase in risk among those who use the pill in their twenties and thirties or between pregnancies. However, those who start taking it when they are very young (under 20) or shortly before the menopause (45 and over) may be at greater risk. The longer you take the pill the greater the risk.

Is hormone replacement therapy (HRT) a risk?

Prolonged use (10 to 15 years) of full-dose HRT is thought to increase a woman's risk of developing breast cancer by about 50 per cent. However, most post-menopausal women are more at risk from heart disease and osteoporosis than from breast cancer, and HRT is currently thought to protect against these.

Does it help to have babies?

Yes, particularly if you have them young. Women who have their first baby after the age of 30 are about twice as likely to get breast cancer as women who have their first before they are 20. Women at the highest risk are those who have a first baby after 35. Women who have no babies at all also run an increased risk. Having babies seems to be protective because it cuts down the number of menstrual cycles you have in your lifetime, and may reduce the number of cells that can produce cancer. Similarly, women who start their periods late and end them early are less likely to get breast cancer than those who menstruate early and have a late menopause. Women who have a natural menopause after 55 are nearly twice as likely to get breast cancer as those who go through the change at 45. And women who have both ovaries removed before they are 35 run less than half the risk of others.

What about breastfeeding?

There is evidence that breastfeeding protects against breast cancer, particularly if you breastfeed your baby for three months or more.

What part do genes play in all this?

Fewer than 10 per cent of all breast cancer cases are inherited, most through a combination of genes which work in subtle interplay with the environment. A few familial breast cancers are linked to mutations in two recently identified genes known as BRCA1 and BRCA2. Women who inherit the fault have an 80 per cent risk over their lifetime. Half will develop the disease by 50 and a few will get it in their thirties. Some women who know they carry the faulty gene opt to protect themselves by having pre-emptive double mastectomies before the illness shows up. For further information, see pages 31–33 and 36.

Is it true that stress makes you more vulnerable to cancer?

Practically everyone believes that stress encourages cancer, but in fact there is no firm evidence to support this.

What about injuries to the breasts?

Women often discover lumps after they have bruised themselves, but this is probably because they rub the tender area and thus discover a lump that might otherwise have remained undetected until it was much bigger.

Can squashing your breasts – as during a mammogram – lead to cancer?

An Australian doctor recently floated the idea that the vice-like grip of the mammography machine might actually cause minute cancerous lumps to burst and spread, turning potentially curable tumours into killers. It seems credible, but the idea was shot down in flames by his peers, who say there is not one shred of evidence to prove that this is happening. Let's hope they are right.

My mother always said that women who get breast cysts don't get cancer. Is this true?

Sadly, no. Women with cysts (or any type of benign breast disease) can develop breast cancer. But they are also more likely to get regular examinations, so they stand a better chance of getting early treatment.

Is breast cancer catching?

No. We now know that familial breast cancer is due to the passing on of abnormal genes. The advantages of breastfeeding for mother and child are overwhelming.

Should I alter my diet?

Some experts reckon that deaths from breast cancer could be cut by half – saving about 7,500 lives a year in the UK – if women changed from their typical high-fat diet to a low-fat, high-fibre one. Most doctors now agree that you can help reduce your cancer risk by increasing your intake of fresh fruit and vegetables, soya and cereal products, and avoiding animal fats (see page 36). Recent trials have shown that olive oil and garlic may be protective.

What about vitamins?

The antioxidant vitamins betacarotene (the precursor of vitamin A), vitamin C and vitamin E protect against cancer, and you should get enough if you eat a normal, balanced diet. Whether it is worth taking supplements is under debate. However, leading expert Professor Anthony Diplock has suggested that, in view of the difficulty of ensuring an optimal diet, supplements would be sensible.

Is drinking alcohol a risk?

Experts disagree. If there is a risk it is small and, provided you drink moderately – say two glasses of wine a day – it will probably be offset by the benefit to your heart.

How about being overweight?

Seriously overweight women past the menopause are twice as likely to develop breast cancer as those of normal weight; for unknown reasons this does not seem to apply to younger women.

I've heard that wearing a bra is dangerous. Is there any truth in this?

The idea that wearing a bra encourages cancer by trapping toxins was recently put forward by researchers at the Institute for Culturogenic Studies in Hawaii. Researchers from more august establishments promptly dismissed it as claptrap.

Can radiation – X-rays, power lines or electric fields from machines – cause breast cancer?

Radiation is a risk, particularly to growing breast tissue. Teenage girls who were exposed to radiation during the Second World War were found to have double the risk of getting breast cancer in adult life, and the rate of breast cancer among Japanese women who were affected as teenagers by the Hiroshima and Nagasaki bombs is far higher than normal. X-rays are known to have a damaging effect, but modern X-rays (including mammograms) use very small doses of radiation, and you would have to have an awful lot of them to be at significantly increased risk. Recent reports from the US blaming X-rays for most of today's breast cancer are thought by most doctors to be grossly exaggerated. There is little hard evidence, so far, to suggest that VDUs and power cables are generally dangerous.

Is there a link between breast cancer and chemical pollution?

The jury is still out on this. One study found that women with breast cancer had about 50 per cent more chemicals in their breast fat than other women. Another showed that breast cancer was more common among women who worked in the pharmaceutical and agricultural industries, and among those who live near hazardous waste sites. But other studies have failed to show any link. Waste products found in rivers and seawater, particularly detergents, are chemically similar to the female hormone oestrogen, which stimulates the growth of certain breast cancers. But, so far, there is no definite link.

Does smoking cause breast cancer?

No. But it will kill you in countless other ways, so don't do it.

This is a revised version of an article first published in *YOU Magazine*.

4

Understanding breast cancer

DR MIRIAM STOPPARD

Of all the different types of cancer, breast cancer has probably been studied most, and we know a great deal about the factors that can increase your risk of contracting the disease. This chapter will help you to assess whether you're in a high-risk or low-risk group, and discover ways in which you can change your lifestyle and minimize your risk. Breast cancer has social, emotional and sexual consequences that will affect not only a woman's health but her relationships, her lifestyle and her body-image. A knowledgeable and well-informed woman is best placed to take an active role in her treatment, and to cultivate the mental attitude that can contribute to the defeat of the disease.

It's important for you to know that, even when a diagnosis of breast cancer is made, there are different types. Not all cancers have the same degree of invasiveness or potential for spread, so not all have a poor outlook. Try not to think of the diagnosis of breast cancer as a death knell. Large numbers of women live comfortably for many years after treatment. A positive state of mind is a real asset, possibly as important as some medical treatments, for we know from research done in Sweden that women who get angry at their tumours seem to live longer than women who passively accept their fate.

Pioneers of treatment

Breast cancer is by no means a new disease; it was recorded by the ancient Egyptians and described by Hippocrates in the fifth century BC and Celsus in the first century AD. A Roman surgeon, Leonides, was known to have operated on malignant cancers of the breast at the end of the first century AD, using cautery (a hot needle) to control the bleeding and scorch any remnant of the cancer. In the same period, the Greek physician Galen set out the criteria for the surgical and medical management of breast cancer, and his guidelines were followed until the sixteenth century. We have come a long way since then. So women over the millennia have been coming to terms with breast cancer and have had to put up with much worse than we do: a letter written by the diarist Fanny Burney to her niece in the eighteenth century describes a mastectomy undertaken without any anaesthetic!

The nature of breast cancer

Breast cancer is a family of conditions, not a single entity. The common feature of every type, however, is that certain cells start to grow out of control. Cell growth is normally restricted to simple repair so that an organ is kept up to scratch: it is held in check by chemicals which ensure that growth is orderly and never gets out of hand. Cancer starts when the brakes on growth are taken off, or when they are no longer effective, or when cells become insensitive to them. Cell growth then becomes uncontrolled and disorderly and the cells themselves may start to look abnormal. Because cell growth is rapid in a cancer, it absorbs a great deal of body energy. This is why cancer is often accompanied by weight loss, though this is rare in breast cancer.

Tumours and spread

Where tissues are solid – as in the lung or the breast – fast-growing cancer cells will produce a swelling or tumour. The word tumour simply means a lump. Most tumours are not cancerous. They are usually benign: the growth of cells is confined to the area where the tumour starts. Tumours whose cells don't spread to other parts of the body are not fatal. In contrast, the cells that make up cancerous tumours are invasive. They spread beyond their original location, not just into adjacent tissues, but to other distant parts of the body, and as they invade tissue they destroy it.

The spread of cancer cells to the surrounding fat, downwards to the muscles, or upwards to the skin, is described as local spread. When cells spread further via the blood or lymphatic fluid, it is called dissemination. The original tumour is known as the primary, and tumours that arise from these cancerous cells that have spread elsewhere are called secondaries or metastases.

The rate at which cancerous cells invade or spread varies greatly: this rate determines how malignant and, therefore, how dangerous a tumour may be. To determine how aggressive cancer cells are and how far they have spread, if at all, grading and staging tests are done. These tests also serve as a basis for deciding on treatment.

Spread through the lymphatic system

Cancers of the breast often drain first into the lymph nodes in the armpits (the axillary lymph nodes), causing swelling. They may also spread to lymph nodes under the breastbone and above the collarbone. (This is why you should always include a check of your armpits and collarbone for swollen lymph nodes whenever you carry out your regular breast self-examination.) The lymphatic system forms a crucial part of the body's defence against infection and possibly cancer. Lymph nodes that are completely free of cancer cells are sometimes taken as a sign of a woman's high natural resistance to cancer. It may only be when this natural resistance is exhausted that the diseased cells break through into lymph nodes. If laboratory analysis discovers that the cancer has spread, this will be considered to be serious and will be reflected in the staging of the tumour, the woman's treatment, and her future outlook. The axilla will need to be treated as well as the breast.

Cancer in the bloodstream

While the first sign of spread may be enlarged lymph nodes, spread via the bloodstream is probably more important in determining the final outcome of the disease. The most recent research suggests that breast cancer cells, or particles of them, enter the bloodstream relatively early in the course of the disease. This is why modern treatments, like chemotherapy, are aimed at eradicating cancer cells from the body *as a whole* rather than just dealing with the tumour locally. The spread of cancer through the blood probably begins with direct invasion by tumour cells of the veins that drain the breast; from there they pass into the bloodstream. These cancer 'seeds' may later form secondary deposits, or metastases, most commonly found in bones or the liver, lungs, or brain. It is almost always the secondary metastases that are responsible for the fatal outcome of a breast cancer.

Fibroblasts

Some research has centred on whether there may be some link between the character of a woman's breast tissue and her risk of developing breast cancer. Recently some researchers have suggested that it may not be the glandular elements of the breast that determine whether cells change from normal to cancerous, but cells called fibroblasts. These lie among the fat and connective tissue of the breast, and produce a number of chemical messengers called growth factors. These growth factors seem to communicate with breast cancer cells, stimulating their growth and their ability to spread. Cancer cells need a rich blood supply to support their rapid growth, and fibroblasts seem to encourage the necessary formation of new blood vessels in tissues surrounding the cancer. It's probable that some women's fibroblasts are more likely to support the growth of cancer cells than others, and this may help in part to explain why some breast cancers are hereditary.

Putting breast cancer in perspective

Breast cancer could be said to be common, as it affects one in twelve women and causes around 15,000 deaths a year in the UK; in the US it affects one in nine women and causes around 46,000 deaths a year. This is not as frightening as it sounds; bear in mind that five times more women suffer from the disease than die from it. In a given year, of 100,000 women who live with breast cancer, 80,000 do not die. More than 70 per cent of women who have operable disease will be alive and well five years after the diagnosis.

Also, with each year you live, your chance of dying from breast cancer becomes less. If you have lived to the age of 50 without developing breast cancer, your chances of dying from it will have dropped dramatically to one in seventy, and the odds get better with every year you live after that without developing breast cancer. This statistic expresses your risk as an individual woman and should not be confused with the risk of a whole population of women.

In statistical terms, breast cancer is the leading female cancer and accounts for almost one in five of all new cancer cases among women. In women between 35 and 55, it ranks as the commonest cause of death overall.

It's only realistic, however, to put these deaths from breast cancer into perspective. For every lump in the breast that is found to be cancerous, ten others will prove to be benign and therefore harmless. Even with cancerous lumps, six or seven out of ten will be treated without the removal of the breast, and for three or four the cause of death will be something other than cancer. If you are prepared to take the initiative so that your lump is diagnosed and treated early, you will be one of the 85 per cent of women who survive for at least five years.

Although breast cancer may be the commonest cause of death in women in their forties, in post-menopausal women – who, by the year 2000, will constitute half of all women alive in the western world – it pales into insignificance when compared with the number of deaths caused by heart disease. In this age group, the percentage of deaths due to breast cancer falls off very sharply, whereas the percentage of deaths due to heart disease rises very quickly. By the time you are in your mid-sixties, your chances of dying from a heart attack or stroke are equal to those of men, whereas your chances of dying from breast cancer are probably less than half what they were when you were 50. So, although the chances of getting breast cancer increase as we age, the chances of dying from it become less with each successive year that we live.

The genetics of cancer

A healthy cell has a well-defined shape. It is a responsible team member and only multiplies when the balance of signals is favourable. Built into cell growth, however, is the hazard of genetic mutations, or random changes. If a mutation occurs the cell becomes damaged and, though it may look normal, it is slightly less responsive to outside signals. As genetic damage accumulates, a cell can become deaf to external messages that inhibit growth, and start to show signs of malignancy. In particular, it loses its regular shape and outline and multiplies uncontrollably. Cancer probably develops because cells suffer irreversible damage to their genes. Events that cause damage to genes are called trigger factors, and those that facilitate cell growth are called promoters.

The development of a cancer cell takes time – it can take several life-times. On the other hand, it can take as little as ten years, depending on how damaged the genes were when they passed from parent to child. Severely damaged genes may respond quickly to an environmental trigger, such as prolonged exposure to menstrual cycling in the case of breast cancer.

Cancer genes

Normal genes that carry messages encouraging cells to multiply are called proto-oncogenes. They come in many varieties – some give cells an internal signal to multiply and others act externally by helping growth factors to stick to cells. These proto-oncogenes can be converted into cancerous forms, or oncogenes. Just one change may be enough to transform the proto-oncogenes, and some believe the damage is a result of mutations. Damage to genes that suppress tumours could also foster cancerous cell growth.

Identifying malignant cells

Over the past twenty years we have begun to identify many of the genes that encourage normal cells to change to cancerous ones. Every one of our cells contains twenty-three pairs of chromosomes and these collectively contain all the genes that form the blueprint for human beings. When dyes are applied to them chromosomes will take up the colour in different places, showing specific regions as a series of light and dark stained bands – a kind of bar code that identifies the individual chromosome. When stained chromosomes from cancerous tumours are compared with others from normal cells, signs of genetic disarray are obvious. Some chromosomes are broken, which leads to several copies of individual chromosomes being present rather than the normal two, and whole chromosomes or segments of them may be missing altogether.

Breast cancer families

A single first-degree relative (that is, mother or sister) with breast cancer doubles anyone's risk of cancer, but in breast cancer families the risks are even greater. A breast cancer family is one in which the risk of developing breast cancer is determined almost totally by family history, and appears to be independent of other risk factors, except atypical hyperplasia.

Breast cancer families, though quite rare, have been studied for more than two millennia and were first reported in Roman medical literature of 100 AD. In the 1860s an American doctor, Paul Broca, described many instances of breast cancer in combination with bowel cancer in several generations of his wife's family. He was describing what we now call hereditary breast cancer (HBC). The word hereditary means that the cancer runs through a family affecting successive generations of women. The pattern of inheritance nearly always suggests that the hereditary factor is extremely strong. The factor responsible has been narrowed down to one or two genes and because it's so strong we call it a dominant gene. Although hereditary breast cancer puts women at very high risk, it accounts for only a small proportion of all cases of breast cancer – between 5 and 10 per cent.

A rigorous approach

There are several important features of hereditary breast cancer that profoundly affect treatment. The first is the early age of onset. Breast cancer is more common in older women as a rule, with an average age of 62 years among women affected, but in breast cancer families the average age is 44. Second, there is often more than one tumour in the breast. Finally, the cancer may affect both breasts.

These three characteristics have an enormous bearing on how doctors view familial breast cancer. Women who belong to these families must be identified and made aware that they are in danger of developing breast cancer early and in both breasts. Any woman who is aware of her risk should seek advice from a breast unit while still in her teens or early twenties. Because of the aggressive nature of this cancer, doctors are more likely to be open to the idea of prophylactic (that is, preventative) mastectomy with reconstruction if you really want to go that far, though medically it's hard to justify when inheritance of the gene cannot, as yet, be proved.

The shadow cast by the hereditary pattern of HBC falls on all aspects of managing it. Monitoring of the health of the breasts must be rigorous and scrupulous with regular check-ups, mammograms, ultrasonic scans where appropriate, and biopsies of any suspicious changes.

Identifying women at risk

At present the most important tool for both doctor and patient is a thorough family history. Unfortunately we have no way of testing for the precise genes and chromosomes associated with HBC and identifying vulnerable women before the cancer appears, though there is hope that such tests will become possible very soon. Until then, a careful family pedigree and close surveillance, with frequent physical examinations and mammograms, are our best weapons. There has been much controversy surrounding the time for starting mammographic screening. The problem with mammograms in younger women is that the breasts are more dense and cancers are difficult to pick up. Several studies have shown, though, that early detection is possible and it's certainly worthwhile in breast cancer families.

Careful surveillance of cancer families is essential. This is best done by gathering the female members of the family together to explain how cancers can run through generations in a family, offering counselling, and subjecting each woman to vigorous screening and testing to detect any cancers early.

Breast cancer genes

Two of the genes responsible for inherited breast cancer were finally identified in 1994 and 1995; it is likely that there are more to be found. These two, called BRCA1 and BRCA2, are probably responsible for more than half the cases of inherited breast cancer. A woman carrying either of them has about an 80 per cent lifetime risk of contracting breast cancer, and a 70 per cent chance after the age of 50. The genes can be passed on by either parent, and there is a fifty-fifty chance that children will inherit them.

At the moment no gene test is available – there are many possible gene mutations, presenting complex problems for testing – but it is likely that within the next five years, women from breast cancer families could be offered a test. Women found to carry the genes would then have the options of increased monitoring to detect cancer early, including annual mammography from age 35, tamoxifen therapy, or preventative surgery.

Excerpted from *The Breast Book* by Dr Miriam Stoppard (Dorling Kindersley, 1996).

5

Breast cancer and western women

DR CATHY READ

The recent discovery that fewer women in Britain are dying of breast cancer is good news. But before we get carried away by this new finding, it is worth reminding ourselves of a few facts: Britain still has one of the highest rates of death from breast cancer in the world, and every year another 26,000 British women learn they have breast cancer. Improvements in treatment and earlier detection with mammography have still had only a modest impact on the overall death rate. 'Magic bullets', modern medicine's preferred solution, have missed many of their targets.

More and more people are asking whether it is time to change the way we think about breast cancer. If we can't cure breast cancer for many women who get it, perhaps we could prevent a lot of women getting the disease at all. After all, prevention is better than cure.

Breast cancer was not always the scourge it is today. Two hundred years ago it was far less common. In some parts of the world breast cancer rates are still low. Women who live traditional lives in the countryside in China and Japan are five times less likely than British women to get breast cancer. These international variations have puzzled scientists for many years. Why should western women suffer more? Investigations into this puzzle provide important clues about the causes of breast cancer.

Imagine you had been born in one of the countries where breast cancer rates have been traditionally low. You would probably have different genes; with no family history of breast cancer you might start off with a much lower risk. Your lifestyle would be very different. Your diet would be less rich, probably consisting of more cereals and vegetables and less meat and dairy products. You would have children earlier, have more of them, and be unlikely to take the pill or HRT. You would lead a much more physically active life. You might also be exposed to less pollution. No one is suggesting you turn the clock back or that you pack your bags and take a flight to China or Japan. In fact, even if you could, you might be disappointed; breast cancer rates are now rising in countries where they were previously low. The global breast cancer epidemic is predicted to claim the lives of one million women annually by the year 2000. Recently, scientists showed that women who moved from Asian countries to the US doubled their risk of breast cancer in just ten years. This suggests that the way we live and the environment we live in may be major factors in determining whether or not we get the disease.

If risks can go up dramatically within one generation, perhaps they can go down again too. This is important because women are often told that nothing can be done to prevent breast cancer. They are told their breasts are as much a mystery as the cancer which can silently invade. But breast health is not a complete mystery. Scientists have spent many years investigating the connections between different women's lifestyles and their risks of breast cancer. Many factors are already known to influence risk, and more are being investigated. They include diet, the timing of pregnancy, breast-feeding, exposure to pollution in the environment, and physical activity. Some risk factors are easier to alter than others, but many raise possibilities for prevention.

Family history

In a 'tour' of risk factors for breast cancer, heredity would be the first stop. A strong family history of breast cancer (where close female and sometimes male relatives develop the disease across generations and often at young ages) accounts for at least 5 per cent of cases of breast cancer. In 1994 one of the main breast cancer genes, BRCA1, was isolated by an international team, and the location of a second, BRCA2, was identified by researchers at the Institute of Cancer Research in December 1995. Geneticists in specialist clinics will counsel members of high-risk families and calculate their individual risks (which are not always obvious and may even be low). Some women at very high risk have opted for preventative mastectomies. Others have more frequent breast screening or have enrolled in the trial of a drug, tamoxifen, which some scientists believe may prevent breast cancer. Scientists are trying to find out how lifestyle and environmental factors interact with breast cancer genes. Once tests for the most common breast cancer genes become available, it may be possible for people at high risk to avoid factors found to increase their risk.

Diet

Some scientists believe that half of all breast cancers could be prevented by the right diet, although there is still debate about exactly what the right diet is. A lot of the controversy surrounds fat. While some experts say women should cut the amount of fat they eat by one half to one third, others claim fat doesn't count. Despite this, several studies have found that women whose diets are rich in meat and dairy products (both major sources of fat) are more likely to get breast cancer. Other foods seem to be protective. They include whole grains, cereals, soya beans and soy products such as bean curd (tofu) and miso, which contain cancer-fighting plant chemicals known as phyto-oestrogens. Fruit and vegetables, particularly red-yellow vegetables and citrus fruits, contain valuable antioxidant vitamins. Cruciferous vegetables – the deep-green and yellow vegetables such as cabbage, broccoli, spinach and cauliflower – contain other compounds which may be protective. The European Prospective Investigation into Cancer (EPIC), an ongoing study of diet and all types of cancer across Europe, is expected to provide even more detailed information about diet and breast cancer. In the mean time there is enough to go on to make positive changes now. It is likely that the best 'anti-breast-cancer diet' will be one that changes the balance of foods we eat: less meat and dairy produce (and less total fat) and more vegetables, grains and cereals, fruit and fish.

Many scientists believe children's and teenagers' diets may be important in determining future breast cancer risk. If this is true, the amount of junk food in children's diets should give us cause for concern.

Alcohol

There is no conclusive evidence that drinking alcohol causes breast cancer, but studies show that drinking alcohol on a regular basis slightly increases the risk of breast cancer. Slight increases in risk have been detected even in women who have as little as one drink per day, and the risk increases with alcohol intake. Some studies have found that young women under the age of 30 are most vulnerable to the effects of alcohol on the breast. Although the British Government considers 2 to 3 units of alcohol a day to be safe for women, mainly because of alcohol's protective effect on the heart, the evidence clearly indicates that this amount of alcohol may increase the risk of breast cancer, especially in the young. Of course young women do not need alcohol to protect them against heart disease – they have plenty of hormones doing an excellent job. Greater numbers of young women are drinking more than ever before; in 1990, 17 per cent of women aged 18 to 24 were drinking more than 21 units of alcohol a week (see also page 48).

Having children

Having children young, particularly before age 20, decreases the risk of breast cancer, whereas having children later or not at all increases it. The average age at which women have a first child has been increasing for two decades. Many women wait until their thirties and even forties before having a child, and one in five British women remains childless.

Breastfeeding

In the early 1990s a spate of studies suggested that breastfeeding could protect against breast cancer. The greatest protection was associated with breastfeeding for three months or longer. These benefits have still not been well advertised. The advantages of breastfeeding are still couched in terms of what is best for babies, rather than what is best for mothers.

In Britain, although two-thirds of women breastfeed their babies at birth, only a third of these are still nursing at three months. Our society is still hostile towards nursing mothers; women often meet with disapproval when they wish to breastfeed in public places, and working mothers find it difficult or impossible to breastfeed at work.

Exercise

Regular exercise appears to reduce the risk of breast cancer. Researchers in California recently found that women who did four hours or more of exercise a week halved their risk of breast cancer. Just two hours of exercise a week, either swimming, jogging, tennis or aerobic exercise, seems to afford some protection. This positive effect seems to work by reducing levels of female hormones which stimulate breast cells every month. This is good news for women – increasing the amount of exercise we take should be relatively easy. Regular exercise strengthens bones, preventing osteoporosis, and also protects against heart disease, diabetes and other cancers including colon cancer. Unfortunately, most schoolgirls and women don't take anything like enough exercise. In 1990, the Allied Dunbar Fitness Survey found that fewer than one woman in three aged between 16 and 74 had taken part in some form of vigorous physical activity during the four weeks prior to being interviewed.

The pill and HRT

The jury is still out on the contraceptive pill and breast cancer; a major review on this subject is being conducted by British researchers. The balance of evidence seems to suggest that women who start the pill before age 25 and continue with it for several years have a slightly increased risk of breast cancer. This has to be weighed up against the benefits of effective contraception and favourable side-effects, including a reduced risk of cancers of the ovary and womb lining.

Family planning advisers recommend that young women are counselled about the risk of breast cancer before they take home a prescription for the pill. Despite the uncertainties, pill-use is skewed towards young women.

In 1989, 19 per cent of women between 16 and 17, 39 per cent of 18- to 19-year-olds and 48 per cent of 20- to 24-year-olds were on the pill.

Doctors still don't know exactly how different kinds of HRT alter the risk of breast cancer. Long-term use of certain types of HRT for ten or more years may be associated with a slight increase in the risk of breast cancer. This has to be balanced against the protection HRT gives women against heart disease and osteoporosis. There are non-hormonal ways of reducing the risk of heart disease and osteoporosis, including diet and exercise; these lifestyle alterations will also reduce the risk of breast cancer.

Radiation and electromagnetic fields (EMFs)

Women's breasts are very sensitive to the damaging effects of radiation. Many women and girls who survived the atomic bombs in Hiroshima and Nagasaki later developed breast cancer.

A question remains over the contribution of electromagnetic fields (EMFs) to breast cancer. Recently, scientists in the US found a small increase in the risk of breast cancer among women exposed to electrical fields at work. A major study is underway in Seattle to determine whether EMFs around women's homes may increase their risk of breast cancer.

Chemicals in the environment

Use of the organochlorine pesticide lindane has been suggested as a link to high rates of breast cancer in Lincolnshire. Scientists are investigating whether lindane and similar chemicals such as DDT could actually *cause* breast cancer. Suspicions were raised after some studies found that women with breast cancer had more pesticide residues in their bodies than other women. It is possible that contamination of animal fat with pesticides is one reason women who eat diets high in animal fat seem to be at increased risk of breast cancer. Other chemicals are also suspected of contributing to the breast cancer epidemic. One group is nonylphenols – chemicals widely used in the plastics industry and in detergents, spermicides and toiletries. Many of the suspect chemicals mimic the female hormone oestrogen. Some scientists believe that chemicals should be screened for oestrogen-like activity before they are released into the environment.

When risk factors matter most

The breasts of teenage and young adult women seem to be particularly vulnerable to cancer-causing influences. Because breast cancer progresses slowly the disease only becomes evident many years after the original damage. Some exposures – including drinking alcohol, smoking, and exposure to radiation – have the greatest impact on teenage and young adult women. Lifestyle changes to reduce the risk of breast cancer will probably have the biggest effect if they are started early. Because of this, research on lifestyle and breast cancer may need to focus on women at much earlier ages.

Protecting women

Putting together the risk factors we've looked at we could summarize what's not going right for women in Britain. Many of us have high-fat diets low in important 'protective' foods like wholegrains and vegetables; many of us have children late or not at all (admittedly a difficult one to change, and fine if it's our choice, but not if women postpone having children because of educational, financial or job penalties); most women who have children don't breastfeed for three months; 'safe' guidelines on alcohol may be increasing our risk of breast cancer; few of us take enough exercise, thousands of young women start the pill early and continue for many years (again, a personal choice to balance against an unwanted teenage pregnancy among other factors), furthermore, we are all exposed to an unknown number of chemicals and other types of pollution in our environment which could be contributing to breast cancer.

Scanning the list, can we honestly say there is nothing we can do to protect ourselves and our children from breast cancer? We might well ask why we aren't being told more about safe possibilities for breast cancer prevention like exercise, breastfeeding and diet. But of course these are not just personal decisions about lifestyle, because our lifestyles reflect the way society works. These are matters for public health officials, policy-makers and the government. While we wait for more much-needed research, let's also ask for action. Why wait when we can start now?

III

The Whole Body: The Whole Picture

Fashion is more geared towards women and therefore we have a ready-made audience. The fashion industry also has an incredible promotions machine to highlight the campaign. Anything we can do to help anyone suffering from illness and disease is well worthwhile.
Edina Ronay

Foods to fight cancer

LIZ EARLE

When it comes to better health, I have always believed that 'we are what we eat.' But can this maxim hold true when it comes to cancer? Over the years, many complementary therapists have drawn a link between diet and breast cancer, despite flak from many orthodox medics. Today, the tables may be turning. The results of many significant worldwide studies indicate that we can indeed reduce our risk of developing certain forms of cancer, including breast cancer, by switching some of the foods in our shopping trolley.

The medical world is waking up to the news that there may be a dietary link to several forms of cancer, and large-scale investigations are currently underway around the globe. Some experts now believe that up to 70 per cent of all deaths from cancer are linked to diet, although the association is not as strong for breast cancer as it is for other forms of the disease, such as colon cancer. As we have already seen, there are many other risk factors associated with breast cancer apart from diet, such as lifestyle and genetics. However, according to Professor Julie Buring, Deputy Director of the Division of Preventive Medicine at the leading Brigham and Women's Hospital in Boston (USA), 'Reproductive patterns and family history only appear to account for a small proportion of breast cancer.' This suggests that environmental and dietary factors may be responsible for many other cases.

In recent years, several controversial studies show that high-fat diets in particular may increase our risk of developing breast cancer. Karol Sikora, Professor of Clinical Oncology at London's Hammersmith Hospital, says 'Looking at all the populations around the world, there is a tight correlation between high-fat, low-fibre diets and an increased risk of breast cancer.' Studies of Japanese women are especially interesting, as their diet has shifted over the last thirty-five years and they are now eating far more fatty foods, such as meat and dairy produce. This increase in fat is matched by a steady rise in breast cancer. In addition, there are more deaths from breast cancer in Japanese cities than in the countryside, where women tend to eat fewer fatty foods. The combined results of twelve studies predict that a small drop in fat intake (around 20 g a day) could reduce the risk of breast cancer by 10 per cent.

Professor Buring is currently investigating the relationship between fat and breast cancer as part of The Women's Health Initiative in the US. Here, post-menopausal women have been placed on a very low-fat diet where less than a fifth of their total daily calories come from fat. We will not see the results of this trial until the next century, and until then Professor Buring and others remain unsure of the link between dietary fat intake and breast cancer: 'We do not yet know if it is the fat, or some other characteristic of women who have high-fat diets, which is the real risk factor.'

To further confuse the issue, not all fats are created equal. Some types, such as the saturated fats found in meat and dairy produce, are less welcome than the polyunsaturates found in vegetable oils. Some studies suggest that eating large amounts of meat may increase the risk of breast cancer – and meat tends to be high in saturated fat. By contrast, the monoun-saturates and polyunsaturates found in vegetable oils may actually reduce the risk of breast cancer. A large-scale Spanish study compared women newly diagnosed with breast cancer with a randomly selected control group. All were questioned about their cooking habits, and those who used the most olive oil had a significantly lower risk of breast cancer. A Greek study, recently published in the *Journal of the National Cancer Institute in America*, involved over 2,000 women. Again, the results indicated that olive oil consumption is associated with a reduced risk of breast cancer.

Unfortunately, it seems that it is not just a high-fat diet that can increase our risk of developing breast cancer. Eating too much of *anything* can raise our risk as well ... Many of the studies linking a high-fat diet with an increased breast cancer risk made the same association with high-calorie diets. The Preventive Medicine Department at the University of California carried out a population-based study of 590 cancer-free women aged 40 to 79. These women were regularly examined, and after fifteen years fifteen post-menopausal women were subsequently diagnosed with breast cancer. These women had significantly higher intakes of all fats, and also consumed more calories than those without cancer. Those who eat large amounts of fat are usually consuming more calories than those who don't, so this link with high-calorie diets may merely be an extension of the connection between too much fat and an increased breast cancer risk. One of the reasons why high-fat diets may increase our likelihood of developing breast cancer is that those who are overweight have greater stores of body fat. This is known to raise oestrogen levels and decrease progesterone levels, resulting in a hormonal imbalance which may in turn increase our risk of breast cancer.

Professor Laurence Kolonel from The Cancer Research Center of Hawaii reflects the common view among breast cancer specialists when he says that at present the link between dietary-fat intake and breast cancer remains 'viable but unproven', although he does concede 'In the mean time there is sufficient evidence of the adverse effects of a high-fat diet on several chronic diseases, other than breast cancer, for everyone to reduce their dietary fat intake.' It is certainly true that too much saturated fat from animal foods increases our risk of developing heart disease – the biggest killer of all. The latest UK *Health of the Nation Report* calls for a 5 per cent reduction in the daily calories we get from total fat. It also advises a drop in those calories that come from saturated fat (from 17 per cent in 1990 to no more than 11 per cent by 2005). Given the astronomic rise in high-fat processed foods, it will be an uphill battle to meet these targets.

Another widely-debated risk factor is the amount of alcohol women drink. Some studies have shown that heavy drinkers have an increased risk, ranging from 40 to 100 per cent. However, other studies have found no such link, and the association between alcohol intake and breast cancer is just as controversial as the link with high-fat diets. As with fat intake, it is not known whether reducing alcohol consumption in later life will minimize the risk of breast cancer. Professor Buring prudently points out that unless proof of a strong link is established, it may not be wise to tell us to give up the demon drink altogether, as drinking alcohol in moderation has been shown to potentially reduce our risk of developing heart disease. As with all things, moderation is the watchword.

Regular visits to the off-licence can be replaced with a daily trip to the greengrocer instead, as we can find much more positive news here. There is considerable evidence that eating plenty of fruit and vegetables has a protective effect against cancer in general. Fruit and vegetables are a complex cocktail of vitamins, minerals, enzymes and fibre – all of which possess important health benefits. In fact, in recent years researchers have focused on betacarotene (the vegetable form of vitamin A), vitamin C and vitamin E for their antioxidant properties. Together, they are sometimes called the ACE vitamins. These antioxidants work by protecting our cells against the free radical damage involved in degenerative diseases such as cancer. Fruits and vegetables are rich sources of betacarotene and vitamin C, while vitamin E is mainly found in vegetable oils, such as olive oil. Senior scientists are currently researching whether it is thanks to these nutrients that fruits and vegetables can protect against cancers. Early results from several clinical trials indicate that betacarotene may be the star protector here. Betacarotene can be found in all colourful fruits and vegetables, especially carrots (hence the name), dark leafy greens, tomatoes, broccoli, mangos, papaya and apricots.

Up until now, the evidence for the benefits of antioxidants has come from both large population studies and smaller trials, where blood samples of women without cancer are taken and then frozen. After several years, a proportion of the group of women examined will develop breast cancer and their frozen blood samples are then examined. The results have been mixed, but some research has revealed that the blood levels of all three antioxidant nutrients, as well as the mineral selenium, are lower in women with breast cancer than in those remaining free of the disease. But before we all rush to swallow a handful of supplements, there has been a great deal of controversy and inconsistency on the subject of antioxidants and breast cancer.

On the one hand, experts such as Dr Rosy Daniel, Director of the Bristol Cancer Help Centre (founded in 1980 as a small voluntary charity aiming to provide holistic help to people with cancer – *see* Directory), put a great deal of emphasis on diet and the benefits of vitamin and mineral supplements in terms of cancer prevention as well as cure. Chemotherapy and radiation increase the requirements for antioxidant compounds, and supplementation can certainly diminish the free radical damage that is associated with cancer. Every year Dr Daniel and her team see around 800 patients with various forms of cancer. They are given supplements containing the antioxidants betacarotene, vitamin C and selenium to protect against cancer, zinc to promote wound healing, and the B-complex vitamins as an all-round boost for the system. Patients are also advised to adopt a low-fat, high-fibre diet rich in organic fruits, vegetables and grains.

The four main antioxidants, vitamin C, vitamin E, betacarotene and selenium, are all readily available from every high-street chemist and health shop. However, the majority of medics remain sceptical about the health benefits of swallowing supplements. Professor Anthony Diplock, who heads the Biochemistry Division at Guy's Medical School in London, is at the forefront of research into antioxidants. He insists, 'We can't jump the gap from fresh fruit and vegetables to antioxidants,' although he remains 'cautiously optimistic' about the future of antioxidant research. It is certainly important to put the health benefits of these nutrients into perspective. Fruits and vegetables don't just contain antioxidants, but also powerful phytochemicals which are still not fully understood. These substances are also found in soy foods, such as soya milk and tofu. It may well be that phytochemicals play a major part in the functioning of some of the body's protective mechanisms, including those which can stop cancer in its tracks.

Health authorities the world over now recommend we eat *at least* five portions of fruit and vegetables daily (excluding potatoes, which count as starch) to help protect against cancer. However, this advice may not be as simple as it sounds. Increasing the amount of fresh fruit and vegetables in our diet may mean that we are also increasing our intake of dangerous pesticides, unless we choose organically-grown produce. In 1995, the government reported that some carrots have been found to contain worryingly high amounts of pesticides, at levels that exceed the permitted maximums. Meat and dairy produce also routinely contain traces of pesticides, including lindane, which has been linked by some studies to breast cancer. Lindane is one of three organochlorine pesticides, the others being DDT and alpha BHC, which have repeatedly been shown to produce over a dozen different types of cancer (including breast cancer) in rats and mice. In 1993, an investigation into the pesticide content of milk in Israel revealed that it contained concentrations of these pesticides possibly 800 times greater than those in the US. Public pressure forced the Israeli authorities to outlaw the use of these pesticides, and it has been suggested that the subsequent reduction in breast cancer mortality rates could be a direct result of this. It is however equally possible that the reduction can be explained by the large influx of immigrant populations, with a lower natural risk of developing breast cancer.

DDT has been banned for some time in the UK, but the 1995 *Pesticide Residues Report* has revealed it is still very much present in some of our food. The report detailed official surveillance of pesticide residues in our food and drink, as required under EU legislation. It found that eight of the seventeen wood pigeons sampled contained DDT, suggesting that it continues to be used in the countryside. In addition, one third of all British chicken livers analysed contained pesticide residues, and 30 per cent of milk samples contained lindane.

A UK government committee recently reviewed the evidence for a relationship between lindane and breast cancer, and concluded that there is no evidence for such a link. However, Andrew Watterson, Director of the Centre for Occupational and Environmental Health Policy Research at De Montfort University, has developed a vast database regarding the link between pesticides and breast cancer. Although the links are complex and, as the government review concluded, not proven, there is considerable evidence from laboratory tests that numerous pesticides, and other chemicals which may enter the food chain, can cause cancer in animals. Dr Watterson raises the all important question, 'Why do we allow the use of these chemicals if we are not sure of their toxic effects, especially when there are alternatives?' He believes that the government should adopt a public health strategy to ban the use of such chemicals, instead of waiting to see what adverse effects they may have on us in the future.

Dr Daniel from the Bristol Cancer Help Centre goes further: 'It is extremely likely that there is a link between high levels of pesticides in meat, dairy produce, fruits and vegetables, and the high incidence of breast cancer.' She goes on to say that the link between high-fat diets and breast cancer may, in fact, be partly a result of pesticide residues in meat fat: 'An increased breast cancer risk could be due to insecticides, pesticides, growth stimulating factors and all sorts of environmental toxins present in the animal fat – and not just the fat itself.' However, cancer specialist Professor Sikora believes that 'Less than 1 per cent of breast cancers are due to pesticides, and the benefits of fruits and vegetables far outweigh any small pesticide residue they may contain, although eating organic is a bonus.'

The subject of diet and breast cancer is clearly a complex and controversial one, but there do seem to be some strong links between what we eat and our risk of developing the disease. To protect ourselves against all cancers, including breast cancer, a low-fat, high-fibre diet is our first priority. Secondly, fruits and vegetables are very high in fibre as well as the key antioxidant nutrients, and have demonstrated a considerable protective effect against cancer. We should all increase the amount of fresh fruits and vegetables in our diet and aim to eat at least five portions daily. It also seems sensible to eat organic food wherever possible, to avoid serving up pesticides on our plates.

An additional option is antioxidant supplements, such as the ACE vitamins, including betacarotene and selenium which may help to boost our protection. However, the link between antioxidants and breast cancer is presently unproven. One thing is certain, though: the foods we eat clearly have a role to play in the prevention and development of many kinds of cancer. This is something that, thankfully, most cancer specialists can agree on.

Vitality eating points

- Aim to eat at least five portions of fruit and vegetables (excluding potatoes) daily.
- Wash all fruit and vegetables thoroughly in warm water with a couple of drops of a mild detergent to remove pesticide residues, or choose organically grown produce.
- Boost your fibre intake by eating more whole grains such as brown rice.
- Avoid high-fat foods such as fatty meat and full-fat dairy produce. Trim all visible fat off meat.
- Drink alcohol only in moderation.
- Consider taking an antioxidant supplement containing betacarotene, vitamins C and E and the mineral selenium.

Additional research by Sarah Hamilton Fleming. The medical trials referred to in this article are listed in Further Reading.

7

Natural breast care

SUSAN CURTIS

Natural medicine is a system of healing based on the idea that natural products will work in harmony with natural body processes. All the processes of nature are interconnected: in order for a meadow to produce sweet healthy grass, for example, the soil must be fertile, the river and rainwater must be pure and the meadow must be managed with an understanding of the natural cycles involved in creating good pasture. For your breasts to be healthy and disease-free, the blood supply, lymphatic and hormonal systems and your overall health and diet must be considered. If your body is healthy you will be in the best position to tolerate treatment and cope with the disruption to your life that breast cancer brings. In particular, you must ensure that you have a sensible, balanced diet.

A holistic approach to health will take into account the need to look after the spiritual, mental and emotional aspects of our lives as well as our physical health. The holistic approach believes that there is a flow of energy between these different aspects of our self, and that this integrates and keeps us whole; disharmony in any one of these areas may push all the others out of balance, and may make us vulnerable to illness.

The increasing incidence of some types of cancer may be a reflection of problems in wider society: many pollutants are considered to be carcinogenic; our western diet of refined, high-fat, low-fibre foods is thought to contribute to cancer; we live in a society that does not always encourage the expression of emotion and the development of a sense of purpose. The fight against cancer cannot just be about finding a wonder-drug, or more sophisticated surgical procedures. We must also address the factors that may contribute to it on every level - physical, emotional and spiritual.

This chapter looks at some natural preparations and techniques which you may find will promote a healthier lifestyle. You can try some of these suggestions, which have been found to help some women. The best way to judge is how you feel. It must be stressed that any complementary treatment you might choose should not be seen as a replacement for conventional medicine. If you have symptoms you are worried about, or if you have been diagnosed with an illness, any complementary therapies should be undertaken only in consultation with your doctor.

Lifestyle and diet

There are many practical steps you can take to improve your health and general wellbeing. Consider whether you want to stop smoking or reduce your alcohol intake (although remember this is *your* choice). Seek medical advice before you take prescribed hormones such as the contraceptive pill or hormone replacement therapy (HRT).

Many holistic practitioners feel that there are benefits to be obtained by changing your diet, and a few generalizations can be made that may be helpful. You may find eating whole foods, including whole grains, beans and pulses, vegetables and fruits, beneficial. In addition, it is suggested that the body will benefit from a reduced salt intake and from a decrease in red meat. So far, however, there have been no trials to demonstrate the advantage of such interventions in either the treatment or prevention of breast cancer. Remember that if you are ill, you need to keep up a high protein and calorie intake. Similarly, the holistic approach is to eat organically grown foods, wherever possible, as you will then avoid the potential harmful effects of pesticides and fertilizers. Unfortunately, such foods are generally more expensive, and, as we have already seen, very little research has so far been done into the possible health benefits of eating organic food.

Several food supplements are referred to in other chapters. Many of these supplements have established themselves in the list of complementary medicine on the basis of years of observation and use. However, few have been subjected to independent validation in clinical trials. In relation to vitamins, it can be argued that if you have a balanced diet, containing fresh fruit and vegetables, it is unlikely that you will be vitamin deficient; but supplements can be taken on the advice of your medical practitioner. Supplements of selenium are popular, and evening primrose oil has been found to help some women with breast pain and tenderness before periods.

Homoeopathy is one of the most popular types of holistic medicine. A homoeopath will take into account all your symptoms - mental, emotional and physical when finding the right preparation for you. If you are considering investigating complementary methods, there is more information in our Directory, but to ensure that there is no possible interaction with other medical treatment, do be sure to discuss everything fully with both your medical and holistic practitioner.

Emotional health and stress

Much has been written about emotional feelings and cancer. Counselling can be of great benefit following a personal trauma such as a bereavement or the loss of a close relationship, and other forms of psychotherapy can be very beneficial in our general emotional wellbeing. It is also increasingly being recognized that counselling has a vital role to play in the treatment of people with cancer; from the time of the initial diagnosis and throughout treatment. This is particularly important with breast cancer, as coming to terms with breast surgery can be extremely distressing for many women. Many GP practices and hospitals are now offering counselling and psychotherapy in recognition of its important role in the wellbeing of a patient. (See Directory for psychotherapy advice.)

Emotions affect our health directly through the effects of stress on the body. A certain amount of stress in our life can be seen as stimulating and challenging. However, dealing with excessive amounts of stress, without an adequate framework for its discharge, can produce secondary effects which manifest as changes in body function. There are some natural remedies that we can use for stress, but these should only be taken at the same time as reassessing the habits and activities in our lives that are causing the stress in the first place. It is useless to relieve the symptoms while maintaining the stressful lifestyle. For example, try to cut down on hours spent at work and add to leisure time; and instead of drinking tea or coffee, try replacing them with herbal infusions of camomile, lemon balm or limeflowers.

Aromatherapy and essential oils

One of the most effective and pleasurable treatments of stress is aromatherapy. Essential oils have many different therapeutic actions, but some of the best research has been done on their activity on the nervous system. Lavender and neroli essential oils, for example, have been shown to have a sedating and calming effect, whereas rosemary has stimulating properties. Combined with massage, essential oils can have very beneficial effects (See Directory for aromatherapy advice).

To create your own calming massage oil, add 2 drops of bergamot, 4 drops of geranium, 6 drops of lavender and 4 drops of marjoram essential oils to 30ml of either grapeseed or sunflower oil. You can massage this in yourself, or ask a friend or partner to do it for you. Alternatively, double the quantities of essential oils to base oil, and add two teaspoons of the resulting mixture to the bath.

Lavender essential oil may be used on its own by adding a couple of drops to the bath when it has been run. As a cure for sleeplessness, add a couple of drops of lavender oil to a tissue and place the tissue near you on the pillow, so that you can inhale the vapours as you go to sleep. Rose is a calming and regenerative oil with a wonderful deep, rich fragrance, good to use if you are feeling vulnerable, sad or tired with life. Add 10 drops of rose oil to 30ml of either grapeseed or sunflower oil and use as an uplifting massage oil, or add a couple of drops of the essential oil to a bath. Several essential oils, including lavender and rose oils, have remarkable skin-healing and anti-inflammatory properties. To make a soothing and healing skin oil to massage in to damaged or scarred skin, add 6 drops of lavender, 2 drops of rose and 4 drops of roman camomile oil to 30ml of either grapeseed or sunflower oil.

Spiritual considerations

Finally, we should look at our health from a spiritual perspective. It is our spiritual self that links us to everything beyond the personal self; and gives us awareness of and contact with the interconnectedness of life. In our western society, with its emphasis on exploitation of resources and material gain, it is very difficult to feel profoundly connected to other people and to the planet as a whole. This has led to very many people suffering from a lack of purpose, and so having fewer resources for dealing with emotional stress and physical disease.

If we can develop our sense of purpose then basically we have more to live for, and we also have more creative energy and joy for life. Finding a purpose - your purpose - is not so much about searching around for what you think fits your expectations, but more a question of identifying where you are now, and what your potential is. Many therapists who specialize in treating people with cancer have observed that those who have a strong will to live and a 'fighting' attitude are much more likely to cope better with cancer. Some women say that confronting disease can be a positive experience. Many survivors of cancer claim that they used their disease to mark a turning point in their life, and as an opportunity to re-evaluate what was really important to them. Cultivating a purpose or a mission can be a part of this process of choosing life.

If you do feel totally in the dark about your purpose in life, it can be helpful to do a life-review. It is important not to become too attached to any one issue, nor to apportion any blame to yourself or anyone else; just look at your life as if it is on a television screen in front of you. At the end of the review, consider what the things are that have given you most satisfaction, such as caring for others, gardening, writing, teaching, being creative or physical exercise. It may be something that you have not done for some time. But if you do realize there are some things that you find particularly satisfying, then commit yourself to finding more time for them. Think about getting out of old habits. Even small changes in behaviour and attitudes can begin to break up the habits and self-imposed restrictions we all allow ourselves to fall into. In our book *Natural Healing for Women*, my co-author and I suggest some exercises for helping to break through old restrictions and patterns.

There are many other techniques that have evolved over the centuries to help us get in contact with our spiritual selves. Meditation is a tool that can enable us to calm the chattering of our brain, and create a contact with the part of our mind that uses symbols and images, and is beyond the rational and mundane. It can help us to restore our contact with ourselves, and with our real needs. Meditation techniques can also provide a kind of deep relaxation that has been shown to be very beneficial to the body in dealing with stress.

Cultivating the spiritual side of your life does not necessarily mean becoming involved in a particular religion. The important thing is to find a group, or a technique, or a teaching, which feels right for you. Being healthy is a process, and you can only start from where you are now and with what resources and contacts you have available to you. (See Directory for further information on meditation, yoga and self development.)

A holistic approach to breast health can bring great benefits, but it is always advisable to seek the advice of a qualified holistic practitioner and to discuss it with your doctor.

IV

If You Find a Lump

To find out that three hundred women a week die of breast cancer in Britain, and that this is the highest figure in the world, is appalling; it is something that we must not and cannot ignore. Fashion by its very visibility can make the difference. Breast cancer is a worthwhile target, and I would be proud to think my small voice could make a difference.
Zandra Rhodes

Human suffering divides into two categories: the avoidable and the unavoidable. With the hope of earlier detection, breast cancer falls clearly into the first. I am delighted to be able to support the fashion industry's initiative.
Nicole Farhi

8

You find a lump: now what do you do?

SARAH STACEY

If you find a lump in your breast, make an immediate appointment with your GP. You may feel very worried but don't leap to the worst conclusion – as you have already read, nine out of ten breast lumps are benign. Your GP should refer you immediately to a surgeon who specializes in breast disease and sees at least fifty cases of breast cancer every year. Make sure you are not referred to a general surgeon who occasionally operates on breasts.

Be persistent: it's your body

If your GP does not refer you immediately, you must be persistent however vulnerable you feel. It is your body. If you get desperate, tell him or her that you will change to a different GP in another practice. The threat will probably be enough, but it is your right to go to another GP and you should exercise it if necessary. Your local Family Health Services Authority (the number is in the telephone directory) will provide a list of neighbourhood GPs.

The experts

The specialist team has several key personnel: one or more consultant surgeons who specialize in breast work, a clinical oncologist (cancer expert), a breast care nurse, a pathologist (who interprets the results of biopsies), plus a radiographer and radiologist who work on mammography (breast X-rays). Your first appointment will be with the consultant surgeon or a senior member of his or her team. Specialist breast nurses should always be available if you want to see one. Detailed notes will be taken of your own and your family's medical history, and then you will have a physical examination.

Early diagnostic techniques

If the consultant finds a lump, a fine needle aspiration will be carried out to draw off some of the cells. (This may be uncomfortable but shouldn't be painful.) If it is a cyst – one of the commonest causes of breast lumps – the fluid can be drawn off there and then, and the problem solved. You may have a mammogram if there is a history of breast cancer in your family, followed by a check-up in a few months. If it's not a cyst, you may have further needle aspirations and certainly a mammogram – again, both procedures may be uncomfortable but shouldn't be painful. Some clinics also use ultra-sound imaging, where sound waves build up a picture of the breast.

From this triangle of information the consultant surgeon and team decide whether they believe the lump to be benign or malignant. In the most efficient clinics you will get the result the same day or within a few days. The British Breast Group (BBG) and The British Association of Surgical Oncology (BASO) guidelines say a woman should have initial screening results (any test) within ten to fourteen days. You should not wait more than four weeks.

If You Find a Lump

If the information is inconclusive, the consultant may suggest a biopsy under general anaesthetic to remove the lump, which will then be tested. The results of the biopsy should be available within a week to ten days according to BBG and BASO guidelines.

If the tests suggest a malignant tumour – in other words, cancer – your next appointment will be with the consultant surgeon, the breast nurse and possibly the oncologist. It's a good idea to take a companion with you. Some consultants will give you a tape of the meeting, others are happy if you take notes. You may want to go in with a list of questions.

Choosing a treatment

Treatment options for breast cancer are surgery, radiotherapy (where X-rays are targeted to destroy the cancer cells), hormone therapy and chemotherapy (where drugs target the cancer cells). These treatments may be used alone or in combination. Each case is different and treatment should be individually tailored. The British Association of Surgical Oncologists has recently produced guidelines so that every woman gets the best treatment. The consultant should discuss all the possibilities, and you have every right to ask as many questions as you like about the proposed treatment and any possible alternatives, side-effects – both short-term and long-term, including possible fertility problems – the success rate, breast reconstruction or prosthesis-fitting service, and arrangements for follow-up after treatment. The breast nurse will be there to give support and information throughout. Although you may feel there is pressure to make a decision, you should take as long as you feel is necessary to consider the options. You may find it reassuring to have a second opinion, and most experts will refer you to another specialist without any fuss. If there is a problem, go back to your GP. Surgery will probably be offered within a week. Some surgeons believe that there is evidence to suggest that survival rates are increased if surgery is carried out in the second half of the menstrual cycle, so you may want to ask your consultant about this.

There are three possible operations: a lumpectomy, or wide excision, where the lump and some surrounding (healthy) tissue are removed; segmentectomy, where a quarter or half the breast is removed, leaving a cleavage (this is usually performed when the woman has a lump under 2 centimetres round); and mastectomy, where the breast is removed entirely.

The lymph nodes will also be tested and possibly removed to look for possible spread of the cancer. The surgeon may also suggest removing the ovaries as a way of treating cancer that has spread. This is a traumatic possibility and patients should question the consultant about the options. Reconstruction of the breast can be performed at the time, but many consultants now suggest patients wait for six months before deciding. Some consultants believe that breast reconstruction is best done by plastic surgeons.

Radiotherapy is commonly given with a lumpectomy and segmentectomy, to stop the disease spreading. There have been revelations recently about cases where patients have been damaged by massively misjudged doses of radiation, but meticulous checking systems are now in place to prevent mistakes. The number of sessions varies but usually falls between fifteen and thirty, given over several weeks. Chemotherapy can be given in tablet form or intravenously, and may be prescribed over several months, possibly starting before surgery. Side-effects may include sickness, fatigue, depression and hair loss. BACUP (British Association of Cancer United Patients – *see Directory*) has a helpful booklet on this.

Hormone therapy, in the shape of the drug tamoxifen (a synthetic hormone) is the most popular back-up treatment for breast cancer today. Tamoxifen seems to work by blocking the supply of oestrogen, the hormone which is implicated in most breast cancers. There may be unpleasant side-effects, but tamoxifen appears to prolong disease-free life, often by several years, to prevent cancer occurring in the other breast. It is also used in cases of recurrence.

Techniques to help you through

Cancer specialists increasingly work alongside complementary therapists to help patients cope with the treatment. All relaxation techniques are helpful. Some patients have found massage, reflexology, aromatherapy or homoeopathy helpful in combating nausea and tiredness; and chiropractic helpful after surgery. A good balanced diet rich in fruit, vegetables and wholefoods, with nutritional supplements, will help to build up the body. Gentle exercise such as yoga and walking will also be useful.

This is a revised version of an article first published in *YOU Magazine*.

My story

MARJORIE SEFTON TALKS TO ABIGAIL RAYNER

I was 48, and although 'too young' to undergo a routine screening, which starts with women of 50, I was lucky enough to have a doctor who wanted to make sure.

I went to my doctor for a repeat prescription for something completely unrelated. While I was there, he suggested an examination. I had no worries about him finding anything, as I felt so fit. I used to be a PE teacher, and I am a naturally healthy person. I was surprised when he found a lump, but still not particularly concerned. It was a week before my period, at which time my breasts can feel uneven anyway.

The combination of a mammogram, ultra-sound and fine needle aspiration all concluded that what the doctor had found was in fact a malignant lump, and I was admitted to hospital. It all happened so quickly I didn't even have time to panic. Within three weeks of my first visit to the doctor I had been admitted to St Charles Hospital in Ladbroke Grove for a lumpectomy and the removal of breast nodes.

I was impressed with the way in which I had been treated, but could not help wondering what might have happened had my doctor not been so diligent. I did occasionally check myself for lumps, but to be quite honest I just didn't have a clue what I was looking for; my breasts did feel slightly uneven but they are glands and one expects that.

I urge women who don't know how to check themselves properly to find out. Go to see the nurse at your local surgery, go to a breast awareness clinic; early detection is so important.

A few days after surgery I had the first dose of chemo in hospital and went home shortly after. I felt incredibly cold and then came down with what seemed like violent flu. Fatigue made me fall asleep a lot and then I'd wake up crying. My mouth was full of ulcers, I couldn't even think about eating because the saliva would cause so much pain. Hair loss was difficult. In the end I decided to have a crew cut, which looked so much better than a thinning patchy mass of hair falling out everywhere. I was a bit apprehensive; I didn't know what the shape of my head was like, but it looked so much better. I was even compared with Sinead O'Connor!

Despite the awful physical side-effects, I believe that the hardest side of cancer is the emotional stress, which has weighed heavily on the whole family. My eldest son Ashley was fantastic; he was the only member of the household at home when I received confirmation of my illness, and he was a tremendous support. Unfortunately Graham, who is younger, did not react as well. I realize now he had panicked about the whole issue. He eventually cried and talked everything through with a friend. After that we managed to move on.

My marriage has been put under strain: my husband found the breast cancer very difficult to deal with and threw himself into his work. He was able to offer little support. It seems that the emotional scars of cancer remain long after the disease has subsided.

Throughout it all, I've had to stay positive. What choice did I have? I have continued to lead an active life, teaching an exercise class three times a week and playing golf. In fact, I've managed to combine my love of golf with some fundraising for BREAKTHROUGH Breast Cancer. I think a way through all this is to get in touch with your fighting spirit.

9

Detection

DR CHRISTOBEL SAUNDERS

Breast problems are one of the more frequent reasons a woman will visit her doctor, and they make up the single commonest cause of referral to specialist clinics in the surgical departments of hospitals. The main symptoms of breast disorders include a lump, or lumpiness, breast pain, nipple discharge, or skin changes. Over 30 per cent of women will consult their doctors at some point in their lives with breast symptoms. The vast majority of these will have simple benign conditions, and once this is established will be reassured and require no further treatment. However, all women should be encouraged to seek help quickly if they detect a problem in their breasts. Since the question uppermost in most women's minds is 'Have I got cancer?', the main job of the doctor is to rule out this possibility and relieve her of this anxiety.

For each woman found to have a breast cancer, nine will have a benign cause for their symptoms. Reassurance that a condition is benign can often be provided by your GP, after carefully listening to your symptoms and examining your breasts (perhaps on more than one occasion through the menstrual cycle). However many cases, particularly older women where the risk of cancer is greater, will be referred to the local hospital. In most instances this will be to a surgeon. This is not because you will necessarily require surgery, but simply because historically surgeons have always been at the forefront of the initial management of patients both with benign breast disease and breast cancer.

A doctor will always start by ascertaining what the circumstances surrounding your symptoms are: how long you have had the problem, the nature of it, and how it affects your life; you will then be asked about other aspects of your health and lifestyle.

Because we know that breast cancer is a hormone-dependent disease, you will be closely questioned about your menstrual history, number of children, breastfeeding history and so forth. You will also be asked about family health history. The more relatives at younger ages who have developed breast cancer, the higher the risk. Age is also a very important factor in the development of most cancers; in general, the risk of breast cancer increases with age. Some benign conditions are more common at certain ages, for example lumps called fibroadenomas, or 'breast mice', are most common in young women from their teens to twenties.

The examination

Breasts vary enormously in size, shape and consistency. It is normal for a woman to have one breast that is larger than the other, some women are said to be 'lumpy', while others always have tender breasts. You are the best judge of what is 'normal' for you. Examining the breasts should include looking at them, in particular with the arms raised, as this may reveal subtle changes such as in-drawing of the nipple or skin dimpling, which may be early warnings of an underlying disease.

Feeling or 'palpating' the breast is done by feeling each part of the breast carefully with the flattened fingers (using the fingertips pinches breast tissue, and so can 'create' a lump). Breast tissue is found right up into the armpit, or axilla, and this area must also be examined. A painless lump is the most common way a breast cancer presents, although other symptoms may point to this diagnosis. A cancerous lump tends to feel hard and immobile with ill-defined edges, but it should be remembered that even with practised hands a cancer can rarely be distinguished by examination alone.

High in the axilla are located lymph glands – these are structures found in many sites of the body which are part of the system of drainage for tissue fluid. The fluid from the breast drains to the axillary lymph glands (or nodes) which may become enlarged as a result of either infection or cancer within the breast. However, enlarged glands do not always mean cancer, and conversely, even if cancer has spread to these glands, they may not always be enlarged. In breasts which are scarred from previous surgery the detection of lumps often becomes difficult.

Women with breast implants are often concerned that these may mask lumps. In fact implants are placed behind the breast tissue, and so any disease which does develop in the breasts should be easily felt.

Special tests

If a patient presents with a breast problem, then the doctor's first task is to exclude cancer. This may be done simply on the history and examination, and if the main problem is pain or lumpiness then no tests may be required. However if a lump (or other symptom such as nipple discharge) is present, it is usually wise to do a 'triple assessment'. This consists of clinical examination, some kind of imaging of the breast – such as mammography or ultrasound – and getting some tissue for examination under the microscope. If the results of all three show the symptoms to be benign, a patient may be reassured. If any are worrying then further tests may be needed, including surgical removal of the lump or, in the case of nipple discharge, removing the duct from which the secretion is occurring. Most surgeons will do their best to diagnose the cause of a lump prior to taking it out. The old scenario – when a patient was given a general anaesthetic, a biopsy taken and, if it proved cancerous, a mastectomy performed there and then – no longer occurs. Women are now given the opportunity to discuss all treatment options before undergoing either surgery or other therapies.

Breast imaging

Mammography is an X-ray technique developed to look at the breast tissue. It involves squeezing the breast between two plates to compress the rather loose fatty breast tissue and so get the best X-ray image of it – this means it can be somewhat uncomfortable!

Mammography can detect a range of abnormalities within the breast, but cannot be 100 per cent specific as to their cause. It is also only about 80 per cent sensitive in detecting breast cancers. It is most useful in women over the age of 40, as younger women have dense breasts which make detecting abnormalities difficult. Mammography is a safe technique and uses extremely low doses of radiation.

Ultra-sound of the breasts is helpful in distinguishing solid lumps from fluid-filled cysts. It is not useful as a general screen, but is often employed in looking at lumps in the breasts of young women where mammography is inaccurate. Other new radiological techniques such as magnetic resonance imaging (MRI) and positron emission tomography (PET scanning) are being introduced, mainly to aid in the diagnosis of difficult problems such as distinguishing scarring as a result of surgery and radiotherapy from regrowth of a tumour.

Tissue sampling

The only way definitively to diagnose a breast lump is by removing some of it for tissue analysis under the microscope by a pathologist. The simplest way to do this is by using a needle and syringe to aspirate a few cells from the lump (fine needle aspiration cytology, or FNAC). This will differentiate cancer from a benign lump in many cases, often within fifteen minutes of the sample being taken. It can be done in the clinic without any anaesthesia – much like drawing a blood sample. If the symptom is nipple discharge, a smear of this fluid can be examined under the microscope.

It does take considerable practice to obtain a good quality sample, and a very high level of expertise on the part of the pathologist looking at it under the microscope. Even then a diagnosis may not be reached, either because the sample is inadequate or because the cells are not clearly of one type or another. In these circumstances a larger needle biopsy is needed to give a small sample of tissue. This is performed under local anaesthesia. Alternatively the lump may be removed by surgery (often under a general anaesthetic). It will then be some days before the pathological diagnosis is known.

Once a diagnosis has been made a treatment plan can be drawn up, bearing in mind both the known extent of the disease and your preferences regarding treatment.

Many women are concerned that the biopsy of a breast lump which may be a cancer will accelerate its growth. There is no evidence that this is the case, and it is important that a diagnosis be made as early as possible so treatment can be planned. On the other hand, there is some evidence that surgery or even biopsy of breast cancers in young, pre-menopausal women during the follicular phase of their menstrual cycle (that is between days three and twelve from the beginning of their previous period) may adversely affect survival. This is being actively studied, but so far evidence is not conclusive.

Many women are also worried about delays in diagnosis and treatment; in fact the growing time of an average breast cancer is extremely slow. It has been estimated that a 1-centimetre tumour may have been present at least seven years since it was a single cancer cell. Therefore what may amount to a few months' delay between initial detection and removal of the lump is not likely to be harmful. Of course, the wait for diagnosis and then for treatment may be very traumatic, and you should have the right both to rapid referral and rapid treatment should cancer be diagnosed. The current aim is for specialist referral within two weeks and operation two to three weeks following this. Breast cancer is not an emergency, however, and it may even be beneficial to the patient to have at least a week or two to come to terms with the diagnosis and formulate any questions regarding treatment prior to surgery.

Other investigations in breast disease

Once breast cancer is diagnosed it may be advised that the patient is 'staged'. This means establishing whether the tumour is confined solely to the breast and/or lymph nodes in the armpit, or if there is evidence of spread elsewhere. In fact, with a small, newly diagnosed breast cancer the chance of distant spread (or metastasis) in the absence of symptoms is negligible. Staging is done with blood tests, a chest X-ray, a bone scan (an injection of radioactive isotope which is taken up by any secondary disease in bones and then detected with a gamma camera a few hours later) and a liver ultra-sound scan (chest, bones and liver being the commonest sites of spread).

Self-examination and screening

Most lumps are found by the woman herself or her partner. Others may be found by routine 'well-woman checks' by a practice nurse, family planning clinic or HRT clinic. While it is most important that a woman is aware of what her breasts 'normally' feel like, including any monthly changes with her menstrual cycle, and that if she does detect any abnormality this is reported early to her doctor, it seems that regular prescriptive self-examination causes more anxiety than it does good. It has often been assumed intuitively that regular breast monitoring through self-examination must pick up cancers at an earlier stage, and thus improve survival in this disease. In fact large studies have not shown this. What does appear to improve the outlook in breast cancer are national breast cancer screening programs using mammography with or without examination. Breast cancer screening has now been introduced into the UK as a population screening program for women between the ages of 50 and 64. These women are offered mammograms at three-yearly intervals (perhaps soon to be two-yearly). This policy has helped increase the detection of very small cancers (with the aim of allowing less radical surgery), and has made a modest improvement in the survival rate. Perhaps more importantly, it has helped to improve cancer services and standardize them throughout the country.

However, the screening program, like everything, is not without its drawbacks. One very real disadvantage has been the increase in detection of the condition known as ductal carcinoma in situ (DCIS). This is usually picked up as a mammographic abnormality which cannot be felt and causes no symptoms for the patient (and thus was rarely diagnosed before the advent of mass mammography). Its significance lies in the fact that it may provide an early warning of breast cancer, and if completely removed is curable.

However, complete excision may mean mastectomy for the patient – a rather radical option when we know that only 25 per cent of women with DCIS will go on to develop breast cancer, and the others will never develop any symptoms of this disease. The problem at the moment is that we do not know which 25 per cent of women with DCIS will develop cancer, and so even though screening has promised saving their lives *and* their breasts, it may not do the latter.

The age limits of the screening program (50 to 64) were imposed because it was shown by a number of studies throughout the world that this age group would benefit the most. Over the age of 65 it is possible to request a mammogram from your doctor. It is increasingly recognized that extending the age limit of the national screening program to 75 may be valuable, as cancer is more common in older women and we now live, on average, to 83 years. Screening women under 50 has not been shown to benefit survival from breast cancer, presumably partly because of difficulties in interpreting the mammograms of young women. However certain groups, such as those with a strong family history of the disease, may be offered mammographic screening as part of surveillance and prevention programs.

Follow-up of women previously treated for breast cancer

Routine follow-up of cancer survivors usually occurs on a three- to six-monthly basis for the first five years, and then annually. This is done in either the surgical or oncology clinics. Regular examination is done, which may be difficult because of scarring from previous surgery and radiotherapy, and the women questioned about any symptoms. Mammography of both breasts is performed every one to two years. If any symptoms do develop these can be investigated with the appropriate tests, much like those used for staging.

My story

REBECCA LLOYD TALKS TO **JULIET YASHAR**

I decided to have another mammogram just eighteen months after my first check-up, simply because I had heard the government were considering dropping this routine policy. Apparently the lives saved by this process had not been significant enough to justify the funding. I thank God for my own initiative. Otherwise who knows; you hear of numerous cases that go undetected.

One week after my appointment I received a phone call at work, informing me that the clinic had discovered abnormal cells in my right breast. My first response was one of complete disbelief. True, I was 54; but I had led a *risk-free* life. I had never smoked, drank very little, ate sensibly and enjoyed good health. There was no history of breast cancer in my family. However, I did not feel anger, or ask 'Why me?' With statistics of 30,000 cases each year in England alone, it's easy to see the odds are against you.

For the first three weeks after my diagnosis, I was totally devastated. I felt hopeless. Breaking the news to my three daughters was not easy. I waited until the result of my test, so as to not worry them unduly. Each daughter reacted differently: one has grown a lot closer to me; another can't get through the day without calling me; the youngest, thankfully, is so busy with college that she is not given too much time to think about things.

My first visit to the hospital went well. I had to have a syringe biopsy, which was rather unpleasant, but not complicated. When the results came, it was not good news. The abnormal cells were malignant, although thought to be non-invasive. I needed further surgery. The tissue biopsy took place a week later, and I was kept in hospital for three days. Then I suffered a post-operative complication called haematoma. My breast doubled in size and became increasingly uncomfortable. The consultant advised immediate corrective surgery before my forthcoming mastectomy. The operation was brought forward yet again when in the early hours of the next morning I had to be rushed to emergency, as the wound had burst.

At present I am awaiting the mastectomy. I have come to terms with losing a breast, only because I have been offered simultaneous reconstructive surgery. To me, the risks involved are worth taking.

My husband has helped me every step of the way. Despite the helplessness he often feels, he is always the optimist, highlighting the positive factors – something I need to stop me from wallowing in too much self-pity. We are now working together, taking one day at a time.

V

Surgery

The fashion industry is probably in the best position to bring people's attention to the cause of women and breast cancer. It is a high-profile industry, with young to middle-aged women as its main focus. This is also the target area for breast cancer. As a 40-year-old woman with two friends affected by this disease, I am aware that it is extremely rampant and very, very scary, both for the women and their families. I hope that by giving this issue a higher profile within the media we can see tangible changes. Fashion Targets Breast Cancer has my best support.
Ally Capellino

10

Operative procedures

ANNA MASLIN & VAL SPEECHLEY

The smaller a breast cancer is when it is detected, the more effectively it can be treated, often using less extensive surgery. In recent years research has shown that for many women lumpectomy (removal of a lump) followed by radiotherapy is just as effective as mastectomy (removal of the breast). Therefore many women do not lose their breast when cancer is diagnosed, although for some women mastectomy may still be necessary.

Lumpectomy

You may need to have only the lump removed, together with some normal tissue surrounding it to make sure no cancer remains. This is called lumpectomy or wide excision. In some instances your surgeon may want to remove lymph nodes from your axilla for examination under the microscope to see whether the cancer has spread to the nodes.

Segmentectomy

This operation is slightly more extensive than a lumpectomy, as a segment of the breast is removed. Lymph nodes from your axilla may be taken for examination.

Mastectomy

When mastectomy is performed all of the breast tissue is removed and lymph nodes are usually taken from your axilla for examination, but the muscles supporting your breasts are left intact. Depending on the type of operation you have, your hospital stay can vary from twenty-four hours to seven days. It is important that you discuss the recommended operation with your surgeon. He or she will advise you regarding the type of surgery required to remove the cancer, as well as considering your view and encouraging you to be involved in the decision.

Breast reconstruction

If treatment involves removal of all, or a large part, of the breast it may be possible for a breast reconstruction to be performed at the time of the operation or at a later date. Breast reconstruction is the creation of a new breast form, and can be achieved using various techniques: an implant which is placed beneath the skin and muscle and which covers your chest; muscle from another part of your body; or a combination of these techniques.

Breast reconstruction is possible for most women who have had all or part of their breast removed. If you have had a radical mastectomy (with removal of the muscle over the chest wall), radiotherapy, or have large breasts, it is usually still possible, although a slightly more lengthy procedure may be required. You can have a breast reconstruction at any age, providing you are well enough.

For many years doctors believed it was important to wait for two to five years after having a breast removed before undergoing reconstructive surgery. This was because of concern that a breast reconstruction might hide a cancer recurrence, or encourage one to develop. However, research has shown this isn't the case, and sometimes breast reconstruction may be performed at the same time as surgery for breast cancer. Immediate reconstruction doesn't mean you don't have a mastectomy – it provides you with a new breast that will be different from the breast you have lost and from the remaining one. Later adjustments are often necessary.

Some women find immediate reconstruction helps them to cope with the emotions associated with the loss of a breast, and to resume their normal life again. If you are interested in immediate reconstruction you should discuss it with your surgeon, who will tell you if it is possible. Some doctors still recommend a delay, particularly if you are advised to have chemotherapy or radiotherapy. There may be a waiting list for reconstructive surgery because of the limited number of surgeons experienced in this field.

There are several different ways in which your breast form can be created. The method suggested for you will depend on individual factors, but it may be possible for you to have a choice.

Subcutaneous breast reconstruction

In this type of reconstruction all the tissue inside your breast is removed, but your skin and nipple are usually retained. An implant is then placed beneath the skin. The scar may be horizontal on either side of the nipple and continuing around it, or lower, in the crease of the breast. The cosmetic result is usually very good. A subcutaneous reconstruction may be performed for women who have certain types of localized cancer. Removal of the breast along with this type of reconstruction may also be offered to women who have a high risk of developing breast cancer, as a preventative measure. However, some surgeons are concerned about problems which may occur later when using this method of reconstruction, as residual breast tissue may be retained, with a subsequent risk of developing breast cancer.

Submuscular breast reconstruction

This is a simple form of breast reconstruction. During the operation an implant is placed beneath the muscles which cover the chest. The scar is usually horizontal or oblique, and in the same place as any original mastectomy scar. A submuscular reconstruction may be suitable if you have a fairly small breast with little natural drop. However if your breast is large or you have had radiotherapy to this area, your skin is unlikely to stretch enough to adjust to an implant of the correct size. This method is unsuitable if you have had a radical mastectomy during which the muscle overlying the chest wall has been removed.

Breast reconstruction using tissue expansion

Tissue expansion makes use of your skin's ability to stretch, just as the abdomen stretches during pregnancy. It may involve two operations, and will take four to six months to complete. During the first operation, an inflatable silicone bag is inserted beneath the skin and muscle of your chest. It is partly filled with sterile saline (salt water) via a valve. Over the next two months the size is gradually increased by introducing more fluid; this stretches your skin and muscle.

The fluid can be added every one or two weeks in the outpatient clinic. This will continue until the size is slightly larger than your normal breast, and then it will be left for three months. During the second operation the silicone bag of saline is removed and replaced by an implant. The implant will match the size of your own breast, and the previous over-expansion will allow it to droop more realistically.

A second method of tissue expansion uses a silicone implant with an inflatable chamber. This doesn't need to be removed from the body, so after being inflated and left for three months, it is deflated to the size of your natural breast. A small operation, usually done as an outpatient procedure under local anaesthetic, then removes the valve.

You may experience some discomfort when the expander is being inflated, and your breast may feel tight and hard. This usually disappears within 48 hours after each inflation. If the discomfort is great, you should contact your surgeon, who may remove some of the fluid and then proceed more slowly with the inflation.

Breast reconstruction using tissue expansion does take longer to complete than other methods, and a few women find this frustrating. However, it can provide good results, and it avoids the need for slightly larger surgery or more scanning.

Tissue expansion is suitable for many women. However if you have had radiotherapy to the area, your skin will probably have lost a lot of its stretchiness and because of this, tissue expansion may not be possible. It is not suitable if you have had a radical mastectomy.

Reconstruction using muscle and skin from the back or the abdomen

It is possible that you may not have enough skin and muscle to create a breast form of the same size as your natural breast by the above methods. This could be for a variety of reasons:

- if your breasts are naturally larger
- if you have previously had radiotherapy
- if you have had a radical mastectomy
- if you have a tight mastectomy scar.

However, in these cases surgeons are able to use muscle and skin from your back or abdomen to reconstruct a breast form.

You have a very large muscle on your back called the latissimus dorsi muscle. Part of this muscle and the overlying skin can be transferred, with its own blood supply, to the front of the chest. The muscle is tunnelled underneath the skin below the axilla (armpit), where it can be joined to the skin and muscle of the chest. A prosthesis is placed behind the muscle. The scar at the front is oval in shape and the scar on the back is usually horizontal, so it can be covered by a bra strap. Sometimes the scar is placed diagonally, and you should check with your surgeon where yours will be. You will be in hospital for five to seven days.

Muscle from the abdomen is a further possibility. The rectus abdominis muscle is one of the muscles of the abdomen running from your breast bone to your pubic bone. An island of this muscle, with its overlying skin and blood supply, can be tunnelled from your abdomen and joined to your chest wall. Sometimes the surgeon can create a breast using this muscle alone, but usually an implant is required as well.

The scars from this operation can vary. There will be an oval scar on the breast, but the scar on the abdomen may be vertical or horizontal. The post-operative discomfort may be greater at first compared with a latissiumus dorsi flap. This is because it is an abdominal operation. Recovery takes slightly longer and you will be in hospital for about ten days.

Nipple reconstruction

If you are having an immediate reconstruction, it may be possible to preserve your nipple. This depends on whether your surgeon thinks your nipple or the tissue behind it may contain cancer cells. It this is unlikely, your nipple may be preserved. A nipple can also be reconstructed. However, this is usually done at a later date when your breast reconstruction has had time to 'settle down'. The surgeon can then position the nipple more accurately so it matches the position on your natural breast. Usually the doctor will advise you to wait for three months before having the nipple reconstructed. This can be done in a variety of ways: by using the skin on the reconstructed breast; by using part of the nipple from your natural breast; or by using skin from behind the ear. The areola is usually created by using a skin graft from the inner thigh, where the skin is a little darker.

Some women decide against having another operation to create a nipple and are happy with just the breast form. Very good artificial nipples, which you can stick onto your reconstructed breast to give an even appearance, are available. You may be able to get artificial nipples from your breast care nurse or appliance officer. If not, they can advise you on how to get them direct from the companies who make them.

After reconstructive surgery

You are likely to experience some degree of discomfort following your breast reconstruction, as you would after any operation. Some women experience more pain than others, and they may need painkilling injections for a day or so after the operation. However, many women have less pain than they expected.

Although your surgeon will try to create a breast form that closely matches your own breast, it is rarely possible to achieve perfect symmetry. If the amount of asymmetry is unacceptable to you, it may be possible to improve it by further surgery. You may be able to have an operation on your other breast, or the implant may be replaced with one that is larger, smaller or positioned differently.

When you are naked you may notice differences in terms of fullness and droopiness, with your reconstructed breast often being less droopy. Your surgeon will try to make sure these differences are not too great. However, if you feel there is a noticeable variation, you may wish to put a partial prosthesis in your bra to create an even appearance. Your reconstructed breast will feel soft to touch but slightly firmer than your own breast. Immediately after your operation it will feel more firm due to swelling in the surrounding tissues. This may take two or three months to subside. During tissue expansion the breast form will be quite hard and tight. It will become soft at the end of this procedure.

Most women have very little sensation in their reconstructed breast. Occasionally there may be sensation in the skin, but often not. If you have a nipple reconstructed, it won't have any sensation. You may experience phantom nipple sensations, but these disappear with time.

Women do describe a diagnosis of breast cancer as a very traumatic experience. Many find it devastating, particularly if the treatment involves the loss of their breast. Breast reconstruction may help you to cope with these feelings of loss. However, you may find you still have 'up days' and 'down days' even many months after your cancer has been treated.

Both the type of operation and your general health at the time of surgery will affect your recovery. Most women are able to take up their normal activities again within six to twelve weeks, depending on their type of work and lifestyle. As with any operation, it may take several months before you feel your energy has returned. Try not to overtire yourself, get plenty of rest, and accept offers of help with everyday tasks such as housework and shopping. Many women feel able to drive within three to four weeks of their surgery, but this will depend on the freedom of your arm movement and the amount of discomfort you experience, particularly when wearing a seat belt.

It is a good idea to get used to how both your natural breast and the reconstructed breast feel so you are aware of any changes that occur. You may prefer to check your breasts at regular intervals, for example in the week after your period or, if you have passed the menopause, at a similar time each month. If you are unsure about how your breast should look and feel, ask for advice. Your doctor will examine your breasts regularly following your breast reconstruction. A mammogram and an ultra-sound scan can still be performed following a breast reconstruction.

Your surgeon will advise you on whether you need to wear a special bra. Some surgeons advise women to wear a supportive garment for up to three months after their operation, to hold the implant more firmly in place and prevent it from moving. You may be advised to wear a bra at night. Other surgeons think special bras are unnecessary and recommend either a normal bra or no bra at all. They believe gravity encourages the development of a more natural droop to the breast.

A silicone implant won't wear out. It will only be changed to adjust the shape, size or position if you lose or put on weight. It is *very* difficult to damage the implant, only a severe chest injury could do this. The implant won't be affected if you go up in an aeroplane.

It is possible for you to have radiotherapy after breast reconstruction. However, treatment would not be recommended immediately after surgery because radiation may delay healing. Your doctor may advise you to wait until after radiotherapy for your reconstruction because of this.

To find a plastic surgeon, ask your own surgeon if there is anyone in your hospital who performs breast reconstruction. If there isn't, he or she may be able to recommend another doctor in your region. There are a limited number of plastic surgeons performing these operations, and it may be very difficult to get a referral. Breast Cancer Care may be able to give you further information, for example regional centres where reconstructive surgery is carried out and the waiting time for an operation. (*See Directory for breast reconstruction advice.*)

The information for this piece was taken from the *Patient Information Series* (Nos 11 and 23) by Val Speechley published by the Royal Marsden NHS Trust.

My story

PAT SUTTON TALKS TO DONNA RICHMOND

I never found the lump myself, it was found through a routine X-ray. Once they had detected something, I was recalled for further X-rays. The whole process was very quick. They did the needle test the same day I was there; I then went back the following week and had a segmentectomy. Shortly after this operation I returned to hospital to try and see my surgeon; he wasn't available and I had to see one of his understudies, who was not able to tell me what was found. I was sent away knowing that there was still something wrong but not knowing exactly what. I rang and demanded to see my surgeon, and thankfully saw him the following evening. He informed me that they hadn't removed everything. My options were that I could stay as I was or have the whole breast removed and get on with my life. I decided there and then to have it removed, and instantly demanded a date – I was not going to mess around. My decision to have the full mastectomy was instant. I did not even discuss it with my husband. I decided that I had too much living to do yet!

I feel very strongly that there is an awful lack of support for women with breast cancer. During my treatment I was given various telephone numbers of support groups, but it was up to me to contact them. It would have meant a great deal to me if someone had called me just to ask how I was. I did call them on various occasions, but often I was left to speak to an answerphone, which is very impersonal.

The chemotherapy which I have just recently completed was bearable, but seemed to last for so long. The actual treatment was daunting, and each time I went I experienced different side-effects, such as an ulcerated mouth, or sore eyes. Fortunately I did not lose all of my hair – it is growing back well now. But, more than anything, I wanted my body back as my own. I felt that I was losing my identity, although I think continuing my everyday work helped me to fight this.

I have found my experience to be a real eye-opener. I did not realize that there were so many women with breast cancer. Since I had the operation, some friends of the family have avoided me on occasions. Some have even gone as far as crossing the road; they are terrified. You certainly find out who your true friends are. On the whole, the experience was not that bad. I was lucky enough to have a loving family around me.

11

What happens after surgery?

DR JANINE L. MANSI

The operation has been done, the breast cancer has been removed. So are you now free of cancer? The short answer is YES, in the majority of cases. Unfortunately, though, the breast cancer can return in some women – either locally in the breast or in other areas of the body such as in the bone, lung, skin or liver. Considerable efforts are therefore made to try and prevent this from happening. The collective term for this is adjuvant therapy, that is, treatment given after surgery to try and reduce the risk of recurrent cancer. The types of treatment available include hormone therapy, chemotherapy and radiotherapy.

Hormone therapy

Many people will have heard of tamoxifen, which has been available since the 1960s. Having been found to be effective in advanced breast cancer, it is now recommended for almost all women after surgery. Oestrogen is one of the female hormones which is largely responsible for the growth of breast cancer cells; basically tamoxifen works as an anti-oestrogen, thus preventing the cancer cells from growing.

Surgery

Tamoxifen is given in tablet form, 20 mg once a day, and is virtually devoid of side-effects. It has been shown to be beneficial in both women who have stopped menstruating (post-menopausal) and those who are still menstruating (pre-menopausal). For pre-menopausal women a change in frequency of their periods may occur, or they may stop altogether. Thus some women may experience menopausal symptoms such as hot flushes and sweating. Weight gain can also occur, but this is uncommon.

Tamoxifen is usually given for at least two years but more often for five years, and sometimes even longer. Long-term tamoxifen use may slightly increase the risk of endometrial cancer (cancer of the womb); thus women who notice a change in, or return of, vaginal bleeding should see their doctor. This cancer is cured by removal of the womb (hysterectomy); in general it is felt that the benefits of tamoxifen far outweigh the risk of endometrial cancer. Interestingly, tamoxifen also has beneficial effects unrelated to the breast cancer, such as protection against osteoporosis (thinning of the bones) and heart disease.

Other forms of hormone therapy are directed at pre-menopausal women and concentrate on preventing the ovaries from working, thus reducing the level of oestrogen in the body. This can be done with surgery (removal of the ovaries, or oophorectomy), by radiotherapy (radiation directed specifically at the ovaries), or medically by using a hormonal agent (the LHRH – luteinizing hormone releasing hormone – agonists). The so-called 'medical oophorectomy' is reversible, unlike surgery or radiotherapy, and involves giving the hormone agent once a month by injection under the skin. All of these methods cause menstruation to stop and menopausal symptoms to start. This form of hormone manipulation can be an adjunct to tamoxifen or chemotherapy, but is not usually done routinely.

Chemotherapy

Drugs which are directed at killing cancer cells are collectively called chemotherapy agents. After surgery for breast cancer these drugs are given to try and kill any residual cancer cells and prevent others from growing. Only certain women will need or be offered chemotherapy – usually younger women, women with lymph nodes under the arm which have been removed and found to contain cancer cells, or women who have large cancers.

If chemotherapy is advised, then this usually starts between two and four weeks after surgery, when the wound has healed. The chemotherapy usually consists of three drugs given in combination; in general the chemotherapy is given by injection into a vein in the arm and takes about ten to fifteen minutes. There may also be chemotherapy tablets to take. The treatment is usually given every three to four weeks for six cycles, thus taking about four to six months.

Prior to chemotherapy, anti-nausea drugs are given by injection, and then subsequently by tablet for as long as is necessary. Additional tablets may also be given to prevent other unwanted side-effects. There may be some hair loss, depending on the type of chemotherapy given, but this can be reduced to some extent by the use of scalp cooling, which reduces the blood supply to the head while the chemotherapy is being given. If hair loss does occur then a wig or head scarf is usually helpful in maintaining body-image; some women really experiment and have a range of wigs, which can be very stunning. It is important to remember that the hair does not necessarily fall out straight away – it usually starts to thin after two to three weeks – and more importantly, it always grows back! In women who are still menstruating the chemotherapy may alter or stop their periods altogether; this occurs particularly in women who would be reaching their menopause within the next year or two. Contraception to prevent pregnancy should continue to be used during the uncertain period. Chemotherapy does affect the normal cells which are responsible for fighting ordinary infection, and so care needs to be taken.

The course of treatment is usually given in an out-patient setting in a specially designated day-unit run by specialist cancer nurses. Together with the doctor (a medical or clinical oncologist) they should provide all the information needed together with contact numbers in case there are any problems relating to the chemotherapy. Many women receiving chemotherapy retain a relatively normal lifestyle; some even manage to continue working throughout. Conversely, some women experience intense fatigue and this can continue for many weeks after finishing the chemotherapy.

Radiotherapy

This treatment is aimed at preventing local recurrence, that is, the return of cancer in the same breast. It is often advised after women have had lumpectomy or segmentectomy, and sometimes after a mastectomy. If all the lymph nodes have not been removed at the time of surgery, then radiotherapy may also be directed under the arm (the axilla) to prevent further problems in this area.

Radiotherapy consists of very strong X-rays, but feels no different from having an ordinary X-ray taken. It is usually started within three to five weeks after surgery, but may be delayed in women receiving chemotherapy until this has been completed. In general, the radiotherapy is given on a daily basis for approximately six weeks. The radiotherapy department is run by clinical oncologists, together with radiographers and physicists. Each treatment is individually planned, and the skin surrounding the breast may have discreet ink markings placed on it so that the positioning is identical every day. Once this has been done the treatment will start, involving lying under the machine for the few minutes each day. Supervision is carried out through a window or closed-circuit television screen, and there is an intercom for direct verbal contact.

Some women experience only minimal side-effects, with a skin reaction at the site of the radiotherapy. Advice is always given on skin care to reduce this as much as possible. If the breast becomes very sore the treatment may need to be delayed for a short time in order to allow the area to recover. The skin may peel, but should return to normal afterwards. Inevitably, that area may be rather more sensitive for many months after the radiotherapy has finished, and care should be taken to avoid the sun.

There has been considerable concern regarding the so-called brachial plexus neuropathy, where women have been permanently disabled following radiotherapy to the axilla after surgery. This can manifest as weakness, swelling, severe pain and sometimes even a useless arm. It precipitated the formation of a group called RAGE – Radiotherapy Action Group Exposure. Investigations into this problem have revealed that many of the cases were due to women being moved from one position to another while having the radiotherapy, thus causing some areas to be exposed to higher doses than others. Fortunately, the incidence of this has decreased markedly since 1987 (1980–86, 41 cases; 1987–89, 7 cases), and with the current awareness should be a thing of the past.

Medical therapy to avoid mastectomy

Over recent years there has been a trend away from mastectomy towards conserving the breast where possible by just removing the lump. If the lump in the breast is large, then mastectomy may be the only surgical option available, but by giving medical treatment such as chemotherapy in younger women (60 or younger), and tamoxifen in older women, the size of the breast cancer can be reduced in the majority of cases. This then enables the doctor to see whether the patient is responding to the treatment, and usually allows a less extensive operation. Once the surgery has finished then radiotherapy is given to prevent the disease coming back in the same breast. In effect this is really just a change in the order of treatment, from surgery, chemotherapy and then radiotherapy, to chemotherapy, surgery and radiotherapy, but it has the advantage of conserving the breast.

The future

As a result of clinical trials we now know that giving tamoxifen to the majority of women after surgery is beneficial and that chemotherapy improves the long-term outlook in certain groups of women. Unfortunately, a large percentage of women are still not offered optimum treatment, and others, despite being given 'state of the art' treatment, still go on to relapse and die of their breast cancer. So what do we need to do now? First, we should ensure that all women with breast cancer have an opportunity to discuss their management with a multidisciplinary team which will include the surgeon, medical oncologist and clinical oncologist, together with the breast care specialist nurse. This set-up is available in some hospitals, but not all, and hopefully will become more and more common over the next few years.

Secondly, women need to know that research on many different fronts is continuing. This may be as simple as how long to continue on tamoxifen after surgery, or more complicated research such as the evaluation of new chemotherapy agents with novel mechanisms of action, new combinations of drugs, or chemotherapy given at very high doses. The more women take part in clinical research the sooner we will be able to improve the treatment and consequently the long-term outlook for women with breast cancer.

12

Living with advanced breast cancer

DR JANET HARDY

Great advances have been made in the treatment of early breast disease, but advanced breast cancer remains incurable. The average survival following first diagnosis of advanced disease is around two years, but some people will live a lot longer than this. It is a challenge for these women, and for those caring for them, to optimize quality of life and support as normal a life as possible for as long as possible.

Symptoms of metastatic disease

Metastasis, or secondary deposit, are terms used to describe cancer which has 'seeded' or spread from the breast to a distant site. The most common sites for spread of breast cancer are skin, bone, lung and liver. Many people think that cancer which has spread to, for example, the bones, is a secondary cancer. This is not in fact the case, rather it is breast cancer which has spread to the bone. It appears that it is the particular molecular 'make-up' of the tumour that determines at a very early stage how it will behave.

The common symptoms of advanced breast cancer will vary according to the patterns of spread.

- Secondary deposits in bone cause pain, commonly in the back and/or pelvis, but radiotherapy can be very effective in controlling this pain. Bone secondaries can also result in a rise of calcium in the blood; this can cause excessive thirst, frequent urination, nausea and drowsiness. These symptoms can easily be rectified by an infusion of drugs called bisphosphonates, which lower blood calcium.

- Spread to the lungs can cause shortness of breath, coughing or wheezing, as well as fluid on the lungs. However, the fluid can be drained off and prevented from re-accumulating.

- Liver secondaries cause swelling of the liver which, in turn, can cause pain and discomfort in the upper abdomen, indigestion, loss of appetite and nausea. All these symptoms can be alleviated by chemotherapy and various tablets and medications.

- Headache, sickness and nausea can be early signs of brain metastases. This may progress to weakness of a limb or difficulty in co-ordination. Radiotherapy is the treatment of choice, and a course of steroid tablets is usually given.

- Secondary skin deposits are not usually painful, but can break down and become infected. There is an excellent range of creams and dressings available to aid healing and combat infection.

- Cord compression is when a tumour mass in the back pushes against the spinal cord and thus interrupts the transmission of nerve signals from the brain to the limbs. This can be emergency because early treatment with surgery and/or radiotherapy is necessary to restore function. Any numbness in the legs, or difficulties with bowel or bladder, should be investigated immediately.

Surgery

We all develop aches and pains from time to time, and the difficulty for women with a past history of breast cancer will be the worry that any new symptom is the cancer returning. This will *not* always be the case, but any new or persistent problem should be brought to the attention of a medical team, if only to obtain reassurance.

Treatment of metastatic disease

Hormone therapy

Hormone therapy is the standard 'first-line' treatment in advanced breast cancer, except in the case of immediately life-threatening disease, when chemotherapy is used as it works more quickly. One example already mentioned is tamoxifen, a synthetic anti-oestrogen that blocks the uptake of circulating oestrogen into cancer cells and therefore turns off tumour growth. Hormonal therapy may result in a slowing down of the disease rather than regression, and treatment needs to be given for two to three months before assessing response. The likelihood of responding to hormonal therapy is about 30 to 40 per cent overall, with the greatest response rates seen in older women (about 60 per cent). The average duration of response is about a year, although sometimes the disease can be controlled for many years in this way.

Chemotherapy

The term chemotherapy encompasses a large number of different cytotoxic (cancer-killing) drugs, usually given in combination either as tablets or injections. Chemotherapy cannot cure breast cancer once it has spread to distant sites but it is very effective in controlling the disease for a period of time and, in some situations, can prolong life. About 60 to 70 per cent of women given chemotherapy will benefit, and achieve a remission that will last for six to twelve months. The disease will then recur, at which time chemotherapy can be given again. The chance of responding a second time is somewhat less and the length of remission likely to be shorter.

The main aim of chemotherapy in this situation is to make the patient feel better, that is to control the symptoms of the disease. It is therefore important that the side-effects are kept to a minimum. Great advances have been made to control many of the side-effects of chemotherapy. There are a number of very effective anti-sickness drugs for example, as well as agents to protect against mouth ulcers and to boost the bone marrow to speed recovery of blood counts. These advances have greatly reduced the need for hospital-ization during treatment and have even allowed treatments to be given in out-patient clinics.

Radiotherapy

Radiotherapy is a form of X-ray treatment often used in the treatment of metastatic disease. It is particularly valuable to improve control of painful bone metastases, for the treatment of skin lesions, and for brain metastases. It is a local treatment (which means it cannot be used to treat the whole body or large areas) and doses have to be carefully controlled to avoid damage to normal tissues. In the context of symptom control, short courses have in many cases been found to be as effective as long courses. The side-effects of radiotherapy depend on the particular area being treated but are usually minimal, with skin changes resembling minor sunburn marking the treated area. Radiotherapy to the head will cause hair loss, whereas treatment of the abdomen or pelvis can result in diarrhoea and nausea. Some patients com-plain of tiredness and non-specific illness during treatment, but this soon resolves.

Palliative care

Pain is the most feared symptom associated with cancer. With modern drugs and methods of pain control, however, pain can be controlled in the vast majority of cases. Painkillers can now be given as tablets by mouth, by injection under the skin, or even through patches applied to the skin. Occasionally anaesthetic procedures, for example nerve blocks, are used to combat particularly difficult pain. There are many misconceptions about the use of strong painkillers, especially morphine. These drugs are not addictive when used for the control of pain, and are extremely useful not only during the terminal stage of illness, but throughout the disease to control severe pain. There are associated side-effects, for example constipation, nausea and drowsiness, but most of these side-effects either resolve after a few days or can easily be controlled. There is no reason why a woman on morphine cannot carry out her normal daily activities, assuming her pain is controlled.

Many of the other symptoms commonly associated with advanced disease have been mentioned above. Coughing, shortness of breath, lethargy, loss of appetite, depression and bowel upset, for example, can all be alleviated or improved with appropriate symptomatic management. Many people equate palliative care with the prescription of morphine to patients at the end of the road when 'nothing more can be done'. This could not be further from the truth. Certainly input from palliative care services tends to increase as the disease progresses, but it should be offered throughout the course of the disease and be an integral part of any cancer treatment, in order to maximize quality of life and control symptoms of disease and its treatment. Today, there is a wealth of expertise available both in hospitals and in the community, which allows women to live well with metastatic disease, and to die with dignity and without pain.

13

Prostheses: what are they?

DEBORAH FENLON

Most women with breast cancer will need surgery of some kind and, for some, mastectomy will be a necessary part of their treatment. Some will also have the option of having a reconstruction. Hopefully a specialist breast care nurse will be available to talk about the various choices for treatment and how to manage practically after surgery. Losing a breast may cause a great feeling of loss, and may lead to a change in how a woman feels about herself. For many women the knowledge that they will be able to present a normal body-image to the world is an important boost to their self-esteem and emotional recovery. The use of external prostheses (or breast forms) is a good way of doing this. Other women feel that accepting the change in their bodies means they do not need to hide it from the world, and so choose not to wear a prosthesis. Every woman is entitled to make the choice for herself, and to a suitable prosthesis should she want it.

A breast prosthesis is a moulded form, usually made of a silicone gel, which is similar to a breast in weight, shape and feel. It can be placed in a normal bra, where it feels very natural; when dressed, it is difficult to tell which is the natural breast and which is the prosthesis.

Using prostheses

Immediately after surgery the scar will be too sore to wear a permanent prosthesis. However, at this stage many women prefer to have something temporary to restore their natural contour; a soft padding of artificial lambswool in a cotton cover will do this, and will be comfortable to wear. Because the pad is so light it does tend to sit very high in the bra, and so may not look very even; this can be minimized by loosening the bra strap on this side and tightening up the strap on the side of the remaining breast. The pad may also move, so it is advisable to pin or tape it into place. These pads, sometimes called 'cumfies', can be supplied by the breast care nurse at the hospital. A permanent prosthesis can be fitted as soon as healing has taken place and the possibility of any swelling has gone. This is usually about six weeks after surgery. However, many women continue to wear the comfy around the house as a lighter alternative to the permanent form.

Permanent prosthesis

The permanent prosthesis comes in many shapes and sizes. The breast care nurse or fitter should stock a choice of styles so that each woman can try several different ones before choosing which suits her best. Most prostheses come in a pale shell pink colour, although there are a few standard dark skin tones available. To get a good skin tone match is quite difficult; some companies will dye the prosthesis to match the individual. There is also a semilucent dark prosthesis available, which takes up the colour of the underlying skin.

Most prostheses come with a cotton cover. The prosthesis does not need to be worn with a cover and in fact clings better to the skin without it. However, in hot weather it can be quite hot and sticky, and the cotton cover helps to absorb any excess moisture. The latest prostheses are being designed with a ridged back so that air can circulate behind them to reduce this problem. Some women also prefer to wear the cover for aesthetic reasons. It can feel quite strange handling an artificial object with such a 'natural' feel. This cover is also a creamy/pink colour and many dark-skinned women dye it to get the tone they want.

Although the prosthesis is designed to match the weight of the natural breast, it can feel quite heavy. Older women or those with uncomfortable scars or shoulder problems tend to notice this more. In this case a foam prosthesis, such as a Rest Breast, is more acceptable, but does not tend to move quite as naturally as a silicone prosthesis. There is also a special lightweight prosthesis available, which has a shell of normal silicone and then a lambswool pad in the centre to make up the bulk. This needs to be worn with a cover to keep it together.

It is now possible to get some prostheses with adhesive strips to secure them discreetly onto the skin of the chest wall. This is not recommended for at least a year after surgery or radiotherapy. The adhesive strips hold the prosthesis very firmly onto the chest wall and so can be worn without a bra. This can give a lot more freedom in the choice of what clothes can be worn. The adhesive strap can be worn for up to ten days. After this time the natural oils in the skin will break down the adhesive and the strip can be peeled away easily. This self-supporting prosthesis can be worn night and day and also in the bath or shower. However, heavy-breasted women may not find this so comfortable, particularly if they do not wish to wear a bra for support.

Partial prosthesis

Surgery and radiotherapy can affect the breast size and shape even when a mastectomy is not performed. Many women find that their breasts are quite dissimilar after treatment and it is difficult to get a bra that fits well and is comfortable. It may also be a source of embarrassment if it is obvious to other people that the breasts are different sizes. A partial prosthesis can effectively fill out the bra and restore symmetry for these women. This is a shell of silicone exactly like a full prosthesis, which fits between the breast and the bra. Once in place it is generally very comfortable and does not move. Most women say they hardly know it is there.

Nipples

There is usually a nipple shape on the breast form, but for women with prominent nipples this may not match their own very well. It is possible to obtain stick-on nipples of different sizes and colours which can be stuck onto the prosthesis.

Bras

It should be possible to wear a normal bra to hold a prosthesis. This bra needs to be well-fitting and of a medium to firm control, so that it provides good support. This does not mean that they have to be plain or 'matronly'. Many companies now make very pretty bras which provide the necessary support. Some women who would otherwise choose not to wear a prosthesis find that they need the support of a bra to be comfortable, and that without a prosthesis they feel very unbalanced. This is especially true for larger breasted women. For extra security to hold a prosthesis in a bra, it is possible to sew in a pocket, or simply sew two ribbons across the inside of the bra cup. The breast care nurse or surgical appliance officer at the hospital will give advice about appropriate bras and proper fit.

Swimwear

The thought of swimming after a mastectomy can be daunting, but with a bit of care it should be perfectly possible to find swimwear that can look very good. It is usually advisable to choose a costume which has an inner lining or cups, so that a pocket can be fitted. A prosthesis can then be worn in the pocket. It is not possible to keep a prosthesis in a swimming costume without a pocket, as water will get between the skin and the prosthesis and cause it to float away from the body. There are foam prostheses made just for swimming, and many women find that a simple temporary prosthesis can be sewn into the lining of a costume. Finding a costume which is cut slightly higher round the neck and armholes can help to hide the scars of surgery. There are also specialist companies which supply fashionable swimming costumes especially for women who have had a mastectomy. Some of these companies will also adapt existing costumes to cover scars, as well as fitting pockets.

Where to get them

Prostheses are supplied, free of charge, for women who have had a mastectomy performed while under the care of the NHS. Most hospitals now have a breast care nurse who will fit them and give advice about clothing, provide information about treatment, and offer emotional support during this difficult time. Private patients will have to pay for their prostheses, but most private health insurance will pay for at least the first one. Prostheses can also be obtained from specialist mail-order companies and some larger department stores. Breast Cancer Care is a charitable organization which can help with information about stockists, and will also help to fit prostheses (*see Directory*).

VI

Fighting Back

Having a very dear friend currently battling with this dreadful and indiscriminate disease brings home the enormity of the pain and suffering it inflicts. It seems appropriate that the fashion community gets together to highlight the scale of the problem and, by the sale of the T-shirts and by producing this book, goes some way towards eradicating it.
Bruce Oldfield

UK National Breast Cancer Coalition

NANCY ROBERTS TALKS TO SASHA MILLER

Nancy Roberts is a radio and television presenter. In July 1991 she was diagnosed with breast cancer. In 1995 she became one of the founders of the UK National Breast Cancer Coalition. The Coalition is calling for a national strategy to eradicate breast cancer.

My involvement with breast cancer began in 1991. I have to confess that I was not a self-examiner, but I was in the shower one day and found a lump. I was obviously concerned about it, but after seeing my doctor and having a mammogram, which showed nothing abnormal, I was told that I shouldn't worry. Those are the magic words that we all want to hear: 'Don't worry.' So I didn't. But then, about a week later, I was watching a talk show on television about young women with breast cancer. All of these women were dying because they had all been to their doctors with lumps and were also told not to worry. A doctor on the show then explained that 15 per cent of mammograms give false results. Well, my hand was on the phone before the credits had rolled. I called my GP, was very persistent, and in the end he agreed to send me to a specialist he referred to as 'the best breast man in London'. But I know he still thought there was nothing wrong. I think he would have done anything to get me off his back. The best-breast-man-in-London felt my little lump and he too said 'Don't worry, this is not breast cancer.' But just in case, he gave me an ultra-sound test. The next day I went back for the results. Once again he said, 'There's nothing to worry about, but just to be sure I want to do a needle biopsy.' So after the weekend I was back in his office to get the results. I sat down and he announced 'The cells are malignant. You have breast cancer.' Just like that. I had been doing a lot of reading, so I had a whole list of questions. I bent down to pull the list I had written from my bag and as I looked up he was looking at his watch. I thought, 'This doctor's not for me.'

I found myself a wonderful surgeon – a woman who worked with a female oncologist. But the problems didn't stop there. I had a lumpectomy and three of my lymph nodes taken out and sampled. The nodes were clear, which was good news, and we celebrated. But a couple of days later my oncologist phoned to say that three nodes was really not a significant amount, and just to make sure I was really clear she suggested that I have further surgery to remove more sample nodes and have radiation of my armpit to clear up any stray cells. Well, there was no way I was going to have more surgery, and I had read that radiation of the armpit could lead to nasty side-effects; I didn't want to have it unless it was absolutely necessary. So I went to a new batch of oncologists to get a consensus about my treatment and ended up not knowing which way to turn.

In many ways, it would have been easier if I was just one of those women who could say 'Just do it, my life is in your hands.' But I'm not. The problem with early detection of breast cancer, although it's wonderful, is that it throws you into a terrible state of confusion. In the old days, you got breast cancer and you had a mastectomy and that was that. There was no choice. Now we have choices and options and decisions to make, which is very confusing, especially at a time when you tend to be in shock. Thankfully, just after I was diagnosed I read a marvellous article in the *International Herald Tribune* about early diagnosis of breast cancer, and how difficult it is for women because there are decisions to be made. The most important thing it said was that a diagnosis of breast cancer is not an emergency. You can take a few weeks to do some research, to choose a doctor whom you feel comfortable with, and choose the treatment that you want. It was a very important lesson to learn.

I went off to the Bristol Cancer Help Centre for a week, because I simply needed a place to clear my head and to be with people who would understand what I was going through. My husband and I were overwhelmed with the terror of cancer, but the week we spent there absolutely saved us. It was being surrounded by other women – and their partners, mothers, sisters, friends – who had 'been there'. We told our stories, we laughed and we cried. It was about being alive again. While I was there, I decided which doctor to go to and which treatment I should have. Those women gave me the support I needed to make that decision. I decided only to have radiotherapy on my breast.

When I got home I tried to find a support group to continue the positive work I felt I had started at Bristol, but I simply couldn't find one near me. In the end, I gave up my search. I took my breast cancer, put it on the back burner, and I got on with my life as best I could.

In the middle of 1994, I made a series for the television programme *This Morning*, called *Well Woman*. One of the episodes I did was about breast cancer, and I found myself talking for the first time about my illness. I told the story of my misdiagnosis, and I told viewers that if they could feel a lump, they must not ignore it. When the series was screened, the switchboard was flooded. Women were calling to say thank you, and that they were going to go back to their doctors. I remember going home on the train that afternoon thinking, 'I've got to do this, I've got to talk more.' It felt like a turning point.

I had always been an activist. In the 1960s I was involved with a group at my university to end the Vietnam War, and in the early 1980s I had been an anti-diet campaigner, but I had chosen not to be involved with anything for a while. I suddenly felt, coming home on the train that day, that I had to do something about breast cancer. I didn't know what it would be, but I knew I was ready.

At the time, some very exciting things were happening in the US. In 1991, three women had got together and decided to start the American National Breast Cancer Coalition. One of their goals was to get the US government to put more money into breast cancer. In the first year alone they managed to divert US$220 million away from the defence budget and into breast cancer. They now have 350 member organizations and 31,000 individual activist members. Because of their pressure, the US government has increased its spending on breast cancer from US$90m to US$500m. They went at it very efficiently. They have representatives in most of the states and they do big press and media campaigns. They run advocacy training classes and they have become the font of all knowledge about breast cancer.

Well, I started talking to people about doing the same thing here. I spoke to Dee Nolan, the editor of *YOU Magazine*, who organized a breast cancer summit where I met the leading breast cancer people. The feeling was that it was time for everyone to work together. While we were thinking about how to move forward, the word got out that I had an interest in breast cancer. In April 1995, I was asked to speak at two different cancer events in one day. It was crazy. Having two events on the same day meant that the press was split between them. I thought this is a waste. We had to join forces. We needed a coalition. In my speech at one of those events I put out the first feelers for the UK National Breast Cancer Coalition. I spoke about the American experience and said if anyone wanted to do the same thing here, they should get in touch.

Fighting Back

In July 1995 I chaired a big meeting of fifty breast cancer activists and representatives of breast cancer charities and women's organizations at the House of Commons. We debated for three hours, and in the end voted unanimously to launch the Coalition here. We then decided that for maximum impact we should have a big launch, to be held at the end of October as the culmination of Breast Cancer Awareness Month, and it should be organized in such a way as to get the grass roots involved. We felt that it was very important that our Coalition should bring the organizations together, but that just as importantly it should be a movement led by women with breast cancer.

I started talking about the Coalition on my Talk Radio UK programme. We got our first bit of publicity in the press, and the letters started to pour in. To everyone who wrote to us we sent a questionnaire asking about their own cancer, asking them what they wanted to see the Coalition do and how they would like to be involved. So, on October 31 1995, in eleven cities around the country, 300 women lined up for a photocall. Three hundred women representing the 300 who die from breast cancer each week in the UK. Each woman wore a runner's bib bearing the slogan '1 in 300'. It was a powerful statement.

In London we had our women lined up outside the House of Commons, evocative of the suffragettes. In Portsmouth, the organizer Christine Vincent managed to get the entire sixth-form of Bedales School to take part in the launch, because their music teacher had died of breast cancer very young, just six weeks earlier. Our launch organizer in Newcastle took her three-year-old daughter along on the day. 'After all', she said, 'it's for our daughters that we're doing this.'

What was truly inspiring is that the women who organized the launch events had no experience of this kind of thing. They were simply women with breast cancer, or women who knew someone with breast cancer or who had lost someone to breast cancer, or who even had just read about breast cancer and wanted to do something. Two of the organizers were in the middle of their chemotherapy when they organized the launch. They said to me later that it was the best therapy they could have had. It got them involved and gave them a positive outlet for their feelings. And that's something we all need. There's nothing worse than being a victim.

From our first meeting in July we had come up with our three goals:

1   Access: that every woman should have access to state-of-the-art treatment, no matter where she lives. In other words, that there should be an end to the breast cancer lottery which means that, at the moment, depending on where you live you can get the best treatment in the world or the worst.
2   Research: we want an *enormous* increase in the amount of money the government spends on research. In the UK, 15,000 women die each year, one of the highest mortality rates in the world, and yet the government is only spending £3m a year on breast cancer research. The defence budget this year is £22 billion, so something is out of whack, to put it mildly. What we don't want is money taken from other illnesses. We do not want a bigger piece of the pie. What we do want is a bigger pie.
3   Influence: we want women with breast cancer to take a full and influential role in all the major decisions regarding breast cancer issues. Women need to have a say in how funds are allocated and what research is done. We should be sitting on all the committees.

The Coalition is about giving women a voice, and taking control, and the time was right to launch it. I had gone from the shock of the diagnosis, to the confusion of the self-education, to getting through the treatment, pulling myself up out of the depression that followed, and returning to normal life and then saying, 'Now I am ready to do something.' So too had other women; because taking control of something like this gives you strength and gives you back your sense of control over your life. You move from wanting to be in control of your illness, to wanting to be in control of the issues it raises.

Now we have got the Coalition started and are beginning to get the breast cancer charities to work together, we want to become the voice of women's concerns about this issue. And we want to end the isolation, because the isolation is the worst. If you speak to any woman who's had breast cancer, there is that frightening feeling that you're alone. In an ideal world, the Coalition will mix support with activism in whatever combination circumstances dictate. The way the Coalition has touched so many women in so short a space of time is proof of how much it's needed. I know that we will have a tremendous impact.

My story

PAULINE ROCKMAN TALKS TO OLIVIA AUGUR

You never think it's going to happen to *you*, but it happened to me in March 1991. It was actually discovered by an amazing coincidence. I was having pains in my left breast, which I ignored or put down to indigestion, or my bra being too tight: silly things like that. In the end I did get concerned, so I went along to the doctor, who recommended a mammogram. It was an absolute fluke that a lump was discovered – in the other breast, so deep it wouldn't have come to the surface for a long time.

I felt panic. Sheer panic. When I get stressed, which is not often, I clean the oven. So I cleaned the oven for a week. I didn't know how bad it was going to be for me, whether I was going to be very ill or whether I was going to be able to sail through it reasonably well. I worried how it would affect the kids and upset their lives, and how they would cope with it; I didn't want to leave them and miss out on their future. I was just determined, 100 per cent determined. I suppose that this will to survive is what has kept my head above water.

The radiographer was already saying that from the mammogram it looked like a malignant tumour. I had complete faith in the surgeon and I had complete faith in what he was telling me. He took the lump out one morning and did a biopsy, so I knew immediately I came around from the anaesthetic. I didn't have any agonizing wait. He said he would do a partial mastectomy, which would mean taking away about a third of the breast tissue, and that's exactly what he did. I started radiotherapy a month after I had the surgery. I had that every day.

I think I've changed tremendously. The experience of cancer gives you a second chance at life: I've had my previous life and now there's this life. It's opened a huge number of doors – doors I wouldn't even have seen had I not had cancer. Coming to terms with it takes a long time; it took me two years until I really started to accept having a slightly different shape, and the scarring. With hindsight I regret not having counselling or joining a support group. I feel that I might have benefited from it. I cycled from John O'Groats to Land's End and walked coast-to-coast across Britain for BREAKTHROUGH Breast Cancer. The walk was the year after I had the surgery and treatment. It was all part of the healing process for me. It was saying to myself, 'Not only am I well, I'm better than I was before.'

15

Terminal cancer

CLARE FORRESTER TALKS TO NICKI POPE

The pregnancy had been wonderful; seven months full of joy and the warm, overwhelming feelings of impending motherhood. Then Clare Forrester first noticed the lump in her breast. She found it, as many women do, when she was having a bath; and although both of her sisters-in-law had recently discovered breast lumps, they were benign, and Clare imagined hers would be the same. The word cancer, let alone death, never crossed her mind – after all, she was just 23.

My husband Peter just said 'It will be the milk' but I phoned up the doctor straight away and he asked me to come in the next day. He seemed to be a little bit worried about it and sent me to a specialist the following day.

She didn't see the specialist, she saw the registrar: 'Silly girl,' he told her, 'go away and enjoy your pregnancy.' Clare dug her heels in and insisted on seeing the specialist – but he eventually confirmed his junior's diagnosis; it was the milk. Fine, she thought. But on her way out of the hospital, a nurse caught up with her and asked her to go back and see the specialist on his own. He thought there was no harm in a biopsy if the lump was still there in two weeks. It was, and it was solid, not a cyst, not milk. Two weeks further on, the lump was still present.

She was told she had cancer at a routine antenatal check-up:

I was told the consultant, Mr Hancock, wanted to see me and that they might have to induce me. It is very hard to describe the feelings you are going through. I was really scared but I didn't think it was cancer. I was just frightened about what was going on, and how it was being done.

Then he told me it was cancer, and he would have to induce me in a few days, and that a couple of days later they would take a portion of the breast away.

The Saturday after I was told I had cancer, Katie was induced. I had my breast operation on the Monday and thought that was the end of that. Funnily enough I really enjoyed the two weeks that I spent in hospital. It was a really beautiful bonding time with my baby. Like all new mothers, I thought it was the best present in the world and I just couldn't stop looking at her.

Her joy was tempered when Mr Hancock told her that she would need three weeks of radiotherapy to kill any traces of the cancer. 'Death still never came into it, or malignancy, the words were never used. I thought it was a harmless sort of cancer.' Five-days-a-week radiotherapy was no big deal to Clare; except for a couple of blue tattoos and a bit of redness, there were no side-effects.

But other, bigger decisions were on the horizon for Clare and her partner Peter, then 25:

They told me that the hormone changes during my pregnancy had caused cancer; they thought it was a good idea if we didn't have any more children. I thought, 'I have one healthy child, some people don't have that.' We talked about it, and my husband decided he would have the snip.

Clare and Peter confronted their situation with remarkable courage and pragmatism. They took themselves along to the Manchester Royal Infirmary for Peter's vasectomy.

The nurse told my husband to get on the bed and take his trousers down. He did and we waited absolutely ages. A young doctor walked in, looked at the notes and said 'We are not going to do this, your wife might be dead in five years and you could have another family.' We just sat there in utter shock.

Clare and Peter returned to their consultant, Mr Hancock. He explained that although the junior doctor had been cruel and had no right to say what he did, the facts were they could not guarantee the cancer would not come back. It made sense for Clare to be sterilized. Less than five months after the birth of her first child in August 1986, breast cancer ended Clare's childbearing days. She recalls, without bitterness, and with just the faintest note of regret edging through her remarkable front, that it had upset her, because her pregnancy had been so wonderful.

I had never been sick, I really enjoyed being pregnant. I was feeling the warmth of having something, another human being, growing inside of me and this had to come along and spoil it. It was spoiling one of the biggest things of my life.

But the news for the young family got better. Clare went for her check-ups every three months, then every six months, and finally, five years later she passed through the magic barrier. The doctors told her she was clear and it was wonderful. Life was back to normal by then, Katie was a happy, healthy child – and her mother was happy and healthy as well.

So in early 1992, when she started getting lower back pain, Clare wasn't really worried as she took herself off to the doctors. A little over-weight, they said, exercise a bit, and Clare remembers thinking 'They must be joking.' The pain worsened and the GP insisted it was probably lumbago. But by April it was so bad Clare took herself off to casualty. She asked whether it might be linked to the breast cancer, but they sent her home for a week's bed rest, telling her she'd be fine after that.

Then one morning in May, she couldn't get out of bed, couldn't stand. She crawled. As she bent down, she felt her spine crumble and such horrific pain that Clare says she would rather die than go through it again. Peter called an ambulance. The hospital diagnosed two slipped discs and Clare spent two months in traction before being sent home. They got her walking – just – but the pain was still there. Clare ended up back in traction.

This time fate intervened. A new nurse arrived and Clare started chatting to her. She'd come from the surgical ward to orthopaedics and had known Mr Hancock.

I wrote him a little note because he had been really good to me. Within a few days he came to see how I was getting on, and a few days after that I was being sent for scans and other examinations.

And that is when she found out she was dying.

127

Peter walked into the room and said Mr Hancock wanted a word with us. I was really worried, because my family were outside. Mr Hancock said, 'I have something awful to tell you. The cancer has come back and it's in your spine. I will be very, very surprised if you last for the next five or six years.'

How does it feel when somebody tells you are going to die in five or six years? All my family came into the room and they were in tears. You are lying on a bed flat out, you can't move and people are looking down at you in tears and your strength sort of comes back all of a sudden, and you start helping them and you try to lighten the atmosphere.

Katie was just six then and Clare and Peter were advised not to tell her that her mother was dying.

She was only a child, they said, she should be able to enjoy her childhood. I didn't feel happy, I didn't like lying. Children are not stupid. They know when something is going on and they are not being told the exact truth.

At times in traction in the hospital, Clare wanted it to end:

I think your mind starts to give up. I was going to die in five years, I was not going to see my child grow up, my parents were going to see their child die before them. You start to give up because those feelings are pushing you down all the time. I knew I was going to die in that hospital. My family were told I wasn't going to get out.

But then her sister visited her, took one look and decided there and then she would move into the hospital. She brought a garden lounger, toothbrush and ten bottles of wine, and told Clare she would get her out of hospital. When

Clare woke she would try to make her laugh. Neither were religious, but they both began to pray. Her sister prayed one day that the following day Clare would wake up and smile and finally eat something. And in the inexplicable way of these things, she did.

With the love of my family, and feeling God with me, I walked out of that hospital with my sister. Doctors tell you the worst because they have got to, haven't they? But you have to keep going.

By December 1992 Clare was not only home, but back at work. Then Clare read about Lesley Elliott. Like Clare, Lesley was terminally ill from secondary breast cancer and also had small children; Lesley had decided to shout from the rooftops that women were not getting a fair deal. Many GPs dismissed breast lumps in younger women. Lesley was adamant that women must insist on having symptoms properly investigated, and not allow themselves to be patronized or fobbed off. Lesley joined forces with BREAKTHROUGH Breast Cancer to raise money for research into the disease. In a moving article in the *British Medical Journal* she said she was doing it for her daughters and because women would no longer 'go quietly into the night'.

Lesley became my hero. When I read about her I felt so selfish. I was not doing anything about it, especially after having been in traction for three months.

Clare wrote to Lesley care of BREAKTHROUGH Breast Cancer, and the organization asked her to undertake media appearances. Clare did, and she began to learn about the disease which has taken over her body.

From Channel 4 *Dispatches* I learned about the suspected link between the pill and breast cancer. It was really too much of a coincidence. Every girl who had started young on the pill seemed to be at greater risk of breast cancer than women who started the pill in their early or late twenties. I was on it at 16. I had no family history of breast cancer anywhere. Then, when I read there was no research centre specifically for breast cancer, which is taking the lives of 300 women a week, I just couldn't believe it. I was so disgusted. I am trying to do this to give our children a future. Three hundred women are dying a week. I don't understand why every woman with breast cancer isn't speaking up about it. Pressure needs to be put on the government.

Katie now knows that her mother has only limited time left.

Her reaction was wonderful, completely the opposite to what I expected. She just smiled and put her arms around me and told me she was very proud of me and that she would raise money for BREAKTHROUGH Breast Cancer. I don't think she understood the consequences. I didn't use the word death and I have always felt guilty about that.

Clare is determined life will go on. She was frightened when Lesley Elliott died, but remains defiant. She can walk, although she has sciatica. The massive dose of radiotherapy to her spine caused an early menopause because it damaged the ovaries, and radiotherapy to her pelvis and back of the neck have left her drained of energy. She has been on sick leave recently, as her employers demanded more time than she could physically manage.

They told me that they hadn't expected me to last this long and my brain is not as quick as it used to be. I just forget things all the time.

Clare speaks of her illness in a determined way, angry that so little has been done to find the cause of breast cancer, to improve treatment and prevention. And she is adamant that she will go on highlighting one simple fact – 300 a week are dying and there is as yet no dedicated research centre into breast cancer. It is what keeps her fundraising for BREAKTHROUGH Breast Cancer, for whom she is now a media spokesperson. There is more to it than that, though. Like many other women struck down by the disease, she is doing it for Katie, her nine year old, hanging on to ease her transition into her teenage years when a daughter needs her mother most.

They have been wrong before and they will be wrong again. They said six months, they said I wouldn't walk again. How do they know I will die in five years? Katie needs me, especially in her teenage years. I am going to be there for that. I believe that anger will keep me going.

We all need Clare's anger. We need it to remind us that women are dying of breast cancer every day – and not enough people are paying attention.

16

Bilateral mastectomy

DIANA MORAN TALKS TO KARENA CALLEN

Known to millions as the Green Goddess, Diana Moran is a journalist, ex-model and television fitness guru. In 1988, having discovered that she had breast cancer in both breasts, she had a bilateral mastectomy. Here she discusses her experiences of breast cancer, surgery and post-operative life, together with practical suggestions on exercise, relaxation and emotional wellbeing.

Discovering that I had breast cancer

When I was 29 I had a partial thyroidectomy, and that was the first time that I was aware of growing lumps or bumps. On reflection, the surgeon I saw was obviously checking to see if it was cancer – but I didn't have any idea. From then onwards I was checked regularly because it was thought that there could be a link between my thyroid and the possible growths in my breasts – I had a number of benign lumps which were aspirated by my surgeon. One he removed by partial lumpectomy. But at no time did I ever, ever think that I had cancer. Nobody in my family had cancer. I didn't know anyone with cancer. I had lived a healthy lifestyle and cancer was something that I just *wouldn't* get. It *couldn't* happen to me.

Fighting Back

One day I was reading an article in the *Daily Mail* about osteoporosis, and as I was now heading towards the menopause I decided that I should find out about it and get a top-to-toe check-up at the same time. I went along to a clinic and I had the normal tests that everyone has to have – blood, thyroid, liver, heart and lungs. They also suggested that I have a mammogram. I had never had a mammogram in my life; I examined my breasts regularly and the surgeon I was under checked them regularly too – every three to six months.

I had the mammogram and to my utter surprise about four days later I got a message saying that they had found irregular areas of calcification. I went back and was given an appointment to see a specialist, Mr Scott, at the Well Woman Clinic at the Cromwell Hospital. I went along in the same frame of mind as I would have gone to have a cervical smear or whatever. While I was waiting in the clinic a girl came out crying from the doctor's room, another woman was upset, and I suddenly thought, 'My God, they're talking about cancer.' Mr Scott confirmed the presence of something other than my usual benign lumps, and told me that he would like me to have another mammogram. After the second mammogram, I asked him if I had cancer. He said that he thought that I did but wanted to see me again. About a month later, I went to the Royal Marsden to see him again. When I went into the room, he was studying my mammogram. He greeted me kindly, asked me to sit down and tried to put me at my ease. He looked through his notes, shuffled the X-rays and the reports in front of him. 'It's cancer, isn't it?' I asked. 'I'm sorry I have to tell you the news you didn't want to hear.' That was Friday the 13th May, 1988.

My cancer was in the very early stages. There were no lumps, but there were extensive areas of calcification in my left breast and some nodules in my right breast that would also need surgery. My first reaction? Disbelief – and despair. I felt sick, but I fought to take control. Knowledge is power, so I asked more questions. How could it be that after twenty years of self-examination, and six-monthly check-ups since the benign lumps had been discovered, that I had full-blown breast cancer? Only two months before, my doctor had given me the all-clear. Mr Scott explained to me that the mammogram shows up cancerous cells before they form lumps. I was lucky, he told me. I started then to think about the practical things. I'd recently divorced. How would I manage? How would I pay the bills, let alone the mortgage? Who would nurse me? Mr Scott let me unburden myself while he listened quietly and reassured me.

He then proceeded to explain in more detail about the cancer and about the possible treatment. I had non-invasive cancer, which meant that it was more widely distributed, but if they removed the affected areas it shouldn't travel anywhere else. Mr Scott then suggested that the best course of treatment in my case was to have a bilateral mastectomy – basically, both my breasts would have to be removed surgically; I would be able to have breast reconstruction after the mastectomy. Some consolation at least.

My physical body has been my fortune, so to speak. What would happen to my career? How would people react when they found that the Green Goddess, supposedly the epitome of health, had breast cancer? And what about Peter, my partner – how would he feel? And how long would I need to recover? I was told I would probably have to stay in hospital for seven to ten days after surgery. Then it would take about six to eight weeks to regain mobility. Strength and stamina, however, were going to take much longer – as it turned out, it took me about a year to get close to my pre-operative fitness level.

The impact of mastectomy

Almost two months later, I was being wheeled down to the theatre at the Cromwell Hospital. When I woke up from the anaesthetic, my first thought was, 'Thank God. I've made it. I've been given a second chance.' Physically, the pain was excruciating but once the painkillers were injected they provided immediate relief. My next thought was to wonder what they had actually done. Because of the fact that I spend most of my life in a body-revealing leotard, my surgeon had suggested that I could have reconstructive surgery immediately. Although there is controversy as to whether it should be done at the same time as a mastectomy, I wasn't aware of any problems at the time, so when I woke up from the anaesthetic and the nurse told me that they had done everything – the mastectomy and reconstruction – my spirits soared. I felt so relieved. As far as I was concerned, they had removed my cancer. But I still had to get through the physical discomfort. While the painkillers took the edge off the pain, they made me feel incredibly nauseous and in a daze. Gradually, the pain began to ease and the nausea subsided.

Three days after the operation, Mr Crosswell, the surgeon, came to remove the dressings from my chest. Even though he had explained fully what they had done, I was terrified. This was the first time that I saw my breasts after the surgery. They were bruised and stitched, and one was minus a nipple. I then had to slip into a surgical bodice to support me and to keep the dressings in place. I would have to wear it for three months. Initially I was really pleased with the way that my breasts looked and felt, and was quite positive. When I was on my own, I cried – not with self-pity but with relief. There were still physical hurdles, though. For the first week, I found it very difficult to sleep. I normally sleep on my tummy, but of course, I couldn't. And I had drains in both sides to drain away any fluid. But I had good news – I was going to be able to go home. And then even better news: Mr Scott, the specialist, confirmed that my cancer was non-invasive and confined to my breasts, which means that it shouldn't reappear anywhere else in my body.

Of course, going home is not the end of the story. It's another beginning. I really have been given a second chance. But I still had a long way to go in terms of regaining my former physical fitness and picking up my career where I'd left off. I also had to rebuild my self-confidence and come to terms with the impact of the mastectomy, even though I'd had reconstruction. When my bandages were eventually removed – after about two months – both my surgeons were pleased with the results. When I got home from having the dressings removed, I also showed my friend Elizabeth; she'd been through it all herself and was incredibly supportive throughout.

When I first saw my breasts, they were still partially bandaged, so I just got an impression of the shape. It was fantastic – I felt like Botticelli's Venus. Like many women, I suppose one of the most anxious moments is when you first show your partner your breasts or scars. One evening as I prepared for bed, I decided to show Peter. I sensed his apprehension, and I felt embarrassed as I took off the corset and looked down. It was bad timing on my part – I was tired and feeling low. I felt that I was ugly and disfigured, and was super-conscious of the cuts, stitches and bruises. I also felt pain. Even though he was kind and assured me that I looked fine, I didn't really believe him.

It took a long time to boost my self-esteem, and I don't think I had fully recovered my confidence until I had to do a photographic shoot wearing my infamous green tights and leotard. Although I still had two breasts, I only had one nipple – and so in terms of photographs, I had quite a problem. The day before the shoot, I was really anxious. I tried all kinds of things to make a false nipple – blue tack, rolled-up sticky tape – and finally found that the best thing was a raisin! Thankfully, after that, someone told me that you can get prosthetic nipples.

Fighting Back

My confidence wasn't totally regained, though, until I made my first appearance on television after the operation. About a week after the photographic shoot, the BBC asked me to come on *Daytime* to do a workout. I thought, 'I'm either going to get through this or I'm going to fall down and collapse in front of everyone.' It's one thing to do static photographs. I was going to be moving, my body was going to be vulnerable. My book was published just after that and, of course, everyone was taken by surprise. The public certainly hadn't known that I had cancer, let alone a bilateral mastectomy. I knew that I'd done it.

Unfortunately, three years later I had to undergo corrective reconstruction surgery. Things had started to go wrong. The prostheses weren't 'settling down', and my breasts became increasingly uncomfortable. It was difficult the second time around. My own tissue had bonded with the implants and had to be cut out. My skin was paper-thin. This time I came out on a major low. And things got worse. Soon after coming out of hospital, Peter left me. I was devastated and in a daze; practically suicidal. After being on such a high, I was at my all-time low. It has taken me a long time to recover. Had I not had my friends, my sons and family and my support group, I would have been lost. I couldn't believe that I had gone through all that and that he couldn't cope, that he couldn't face me. And I know I'm not alone, that other women have had to deal with this too. Thankfully, I have masses of inner strength, coupled with support, so I did get through it.

OK, so I've lost a lot of feeling in my breasts and one nipple too – so what? I've got my life and my health. It's a small price to pay. I know that I made the right decision. To go through life waiting for changes to occur in the cancer would have made me a nervous wreck. As it is, I can put it behind me and get on with living.

Post-operative lifestyle

As Diana's story illustrates, undergoing a mastectomy takes both an emotional and physical toll on mind and body. But being prepared and being armed with knowledge will ensure that you feel as much in control as possible. One of the most important things is to prepare yourself for the likelihood of external changes in your life, and of changes in the way you feel about yourself.

The side-effects after a mastectomy are different for every woman. Physically you may experience a number of feelings, such as phantom pain – a sensation where you feel that your breast is still there. If you have had one breast removed, it may take a while to get used to the feeling of lopsidedness. And you will also find that your mobility is restricted in the first few weeks after surgery. But there are solutions. Physiotherapy will improve arm and chest muscle strength, and help you to ease gently back into an active life. Gentle, controlled exercise also stimulates blood flow and lymph circulation, which should speed up the body's natural healing process.

For the majority of women, losing a breast can also trigger a host of emotions, from depression to anger. Even if you think that you are Super-woman, post-operative counselling is essential. It is completely natural to go through dramatic mood swings after breast surgery. Some women come out on a high, relieved that their cancer has gone, only to find that they crash down later, just when they're not expecting it. Others come out on a low and find that it takes months to reach a point of emotional stability. Whatever the experience, there are a number of organizations that offer support and counselling (*see Directory*). Many women have also found creative outlets such as art therapy or diary-writing extremely helpful (again, *see Directory*).

Your family and your partner may also need counselling. Initially, many partners may find it difficult to cope with the depression and loss of self-esteem women often suffer in the post-operative period. There are organizations who offer counselling to partners. On the other hand, don't presume that your partner won't be able to cope or won't be able to adjust to the fact that you have lost a breast/breasts. Allow people to support you when you need it; you will find that you recover all the sooner.

Getting fit again

Immediately after the operation you will have to cope with physical changes, from discomfort to restricted movement. In addition to specific physiotherapy exercises, you will also be advised on looking after your arm and hand on the operated side; if you have had a bilateral mastectomy, you will need to apply this to both arms and hands. After surgery and radiotherapy, your arms may become swollen due to a condition called lymphoedema, particularly if your axillary lymph nodes have been removed. Taking it easy will decrease your risk of developing it; this means avoiding lifting heavy objects and strenuous household chores such as vacuuming. Should you experience swelling, keep your arm/arms above your head – at night you can rest them on a pillow. 'Most hospitals now have a physiotherapist or a breast care nurse who can show you specific gentle exercises to do to reduce the risk of lymphoedema,' says Debbie Fenlon, Senior Clinical Nurse at the Royal Marsden, London. 'If you do opt for private health care, you may find that this service is not automatically available – so it's a good idea to ask to see a physiotherapist or breast care nurse afterwards.'

Even though you will be advised to take it easy for at least three months, that doesn't mean that you should avoid exercise. If you have been a regular exerciser, you will have to build up your exercise programme gently and gradually. If you haven't been physically active, you may want to take up some form of activity to help you refocus your life and to get and stay fit.

Except when you're swimming, always wear a support corset or sports bra. Diana Moran found she had to relearn how to use her upper body:

It takes a few months to regain all the movement, and one has to proceed with caution and care. Don't throw yourself into exercise, just take your time and take it easy. The main thing to remember is what I call the three S's of exercise – strength, stamina and suppleness. You need to work simultaneously on all three aspects in order to restore your own fitness level. I started very gradually on my arms, shoulders and chest by gently 'creeping' my fingers up the wall. For the first few weeks after surgery you are advised not to lift your arms above shoulder height to avoid any stress on the muscles and tissues and on the stitches. But you can gently and slowly start to 'open up' your chest – there is a natural tendency to literally wrap your arms around yourself to 'protect' the chest area and to round your shoulders. Gentle shoulder rolls and shrugs can really help to restore joint mobility. Just remember – do everything gradually.

In order to build up your strength and stamina, you'll need to do some cardiovascular activity. Walking and swimming are both perfect. I combine a daily walk with regular swims – I do about ten lengths. Swimming is incredibly therapeutic, and as the water supports your body weight it is less strenuous than other forms of exercise. Again, build up slowly. Start with a gentle doggy paddle and move up to a smooth breast stroke – I wouldn't advise the crawl until much later.

Stretches will help to restore suppleness and flexibility. When you do a stretch, just hold it for four or five seconds – never bounce. You must be patient with yourself. And if you find that your self-motivation is low, why not join forces with someone else so that you have a training partner? I found it invaluable to go walking with somebody. It also gave me an opportunity to talk about things that I might not have discussed face-to-face with anyone.

Post-mastectomy care

In addition to regaining movement, your surgeon or breast care nurse will also offer advice on looking after your chest to encourage the healing process. Wearing a surgical corset or bra will help to ensure that your breasts are supported. You may be advised to massage in skin-softeners such as calendula cream and vitamin E oil to promote healing, although this may not be appropriate for those undergoing radiotherapy. Massage can also help to reduce the risk of lymphoedema and, in some cases, a technique known as manual lymphatic drainage (MLD) had been found to be especially beneficial. In addition to massage, some hospitals have introduced aromatherapy – a form of massage which incorporates the use of plant and flower essential oils – to their programme of post-operative care. Do check, however, with your surgeon or with the breast care nurse before you use aromatherapy oils.

Massage is a wonderful way to boost feelings of wellbeing. While initially you may not want anyone else touching your chest, particularly if you have had radical mastectomy, encouraging your partner or a friend to massage you, even if it's just your hands and feet, will slowly help you to build up your self-esteem again. Self-massage will also help you to become familiar with your own body again. You may be too scared or distressed to look at yourself after surgery, but many women find that self-massage can help to soothe their anxieties and build up self-confidence.

Emotional wellbeing

Diana Moran came out of hospital on a high of relief:

But I came crashing down later. I can't stress enough the importance of talking to people. Especially people who've been through breast surgery. You'll find that you are not alone. It can really help you if you're going through a sticky patch. There are more and more support groups, including ones for partners. I found that it helped me to talk with other women, sharing my experiences. Even though every outcome is different in every case, it's incredibly reassuring to know and to talk to someone who has been through what you are going through.

In addition to the motivation that getting fit again gave me, I also found motivation and support through the church. When I was feeling low, especially at the weekends, going to church on Sunday not only gave me a reason to get up and get dressed to go out, but I knew that I would have the spiritual support of everyone there.

My family, of course, helped me through too. Although initially one of my sons couldn't really deal with my having breast cancer, I found that when I really needed them, they were there. And just having them around gave me a sense of purpose too. When I was first told that I had cancer, I had a great desire to sort things out and to 'tidy up' my family. I wanted to see my two sons settled down and sorted out. I really wanted to get my house in order, as it were. After my second reconstruction, the news that one of my sons was going to be a father was enormously uplifting. My granddaughter Charlotte really has been a great source of joy.

Diana Moran's diary of her experiences, *A More Difficult Exercise*, is published by Bloomsbury.

My story

ANNE CLARK TALKS TO LIZ REID

I found a lump five years ago, when I was 34. I used to examine my breasts quite often on the advice of the family planning clinic. When I found a very small lump I rang up my doctor straight away. He though it might be a cyst and sent me to the hospital, where I had a mammogram. They removed what they still thought was a cyst. But only two weeks later they called me back in, so I thought something was up. They explained that they had found cancer, and gave me the choice of a mastectomy or just having the small area taken away. Because I had two young children they thought that a full mastectomy was the best course to take.

By the time I got home the hospital was already on the phone. They wanted me in at six the next morning, so I didn't really have time to think about it. The consultant tried to explain the different stages and why it was good for me to go the whole way. It's quite difficult to take it in, all in one go. I thought 'It's here, I've got to deal with it.' There wasn't really any time for counselling before. After the operation, a sister from another cancer ward came down and spoke to my husband and me for half an hour, but it was more a case of 'When you want any information you should go to the surgical centre.' She gave me her phone number in case I panicked, but I didn't need to use it. They checked my lymph glands and everything was alright. I didn't have to have chemo or radiotherapy, in fact I was in and out in five days.

Six weeks later, I was back for a normal check-up. They asked me if I had any questions; I think I asked when I could get back to work! It was down to my positive attitude. I was determined that whatever was going to happen, it wasn't going to stop me. I'm quite a busy person rushing around with the children. My son was 11 and my daughter was about eight. She was too young to know, but now I'm trying to break it to her without frightening her – my mother has since had breast cancer, so my daughter could be at risk.

They say you are safe after about five years, which I have now passed, but I've got a friend who had a recurrence after nine years. Once you've had it you might have it again, but then again you might not. I wasn't going to let it get me down. You can't go through life worrying that it's going to come back, you have to cope with what life throws at you. After all, you could walk out tomorrow and get run over by a bus. A positive attitude is the most important thing.

Feelings

The fashion industry is guilty of promoting the perfect woman. Here is a moment for us to show compassion and understanding for all women. Breast cancer is an exceptionally frightening illness and I would like to help make a difference.
Paul Costelloe

Talking things through

LINDA BENN & CLARE CROMBIE

Over the years as head of BACUP's (British Association of Cancer United Patients) cancer counselling services in London and Glasgow, I have listened to many hundreds of women tell me about their breast cancer. There are several key areas which cause stress over and over; if unchecked, this stress can grow and lead to other problems. We all face stress in our lives, often accumulating problems and anxieties as we go along. New stresses are added to old. Thus, the particular worries that come with breast cancer are stacked on a foundation of our own individual histories and life stories; breast cancer stresses begin long before diagnosis.

In the period leading up to diagnosis there are many questions: Is this lump real? Is it malignant? Then there is the shock of the diagnosis itself: Why me? What have I done to deserve this? This is followed by the treatments, the post-operative period, and more worry: Will everyone expect me to be the old me? Will I never look the same again? Then there are the check-ups: Has it come back? How will I cope a second or third time? These stresses, potential and actual, can seem never-ending, especially when the cancer, the trigger, lies beyond our control.

One way of looking at stress is as the suppression of the body's natural 'fight or flight' reaction. When a woman is told she has breast cancer she has to face the fact that the danger lies within her own body; escape is impossible. This danger is compounded by the silence and stigma which surrounds the disease, indeed the very word 'cancer'.

There is a lot of silence attached to cancer. The cancer, for many, grew silently and unnoticed. And the silence continues with people around you, sometimes including the doctors and nurses, who seem to have problems talking about cancer openly and honestly. Even good friends stay away from you, and nobody, it seems, wants to share your cancer experience. When faced with all this, what are you to do with the natural impulse of escape and flight?

Flight can come in different forms, and one of the best known is denial. Others decide that if flight isn't possible, then fight is. Becoming as active as possible in getting well again is part of the fight. A woman's attitude towards her illness, treatment and the people around her, including the medical staff, can enhance the need to fight. This is a healthy aggression.

When any of us feels out of control and is having to deal with internal and sometimes external chaos, anger is to be expected. Anger in women is viewed by society as something destructive which needs to be suppressed. This can mean that women themselves are not aware of their anger. Betty came for counselling at BACUP when her treatment was over. Her doctor had said she was better and she finally had the energy to return to work. Yet she felt she was 'falling apart'.

When Betty began to talk about what had happened since she first found the lump in her breast, she began to uncover feelings she had unintentionally denied herself at the time. She had felt very frightened, and asked herself many questions: Will I die? What if it comes back? How will I know? Will I still be lovable? Will I be able to have more children? Will I ever have a partner who will find me attractive? She couldn't talk about these things for fear of upsetting others. She began to realize the anger she had felt at certain points, such as when the surgeon told her he had done a 'beautiful job' on her breast, and all she could think about was the large part of her which was missing when the lump had felt so small. 'How could you say it's beautiful?' At the time she chose to deny her genuine feelings: 'After all, the doctor was only doing his job, and he had saved my life.'

If the anger, which is a natural part of loss and adjustment, finds no direct expression, we may turn it inwards where it becomes depression, tiredness, loss of motivation or hopelessness. Equally it can turn outwards in a destructive way. A woman wanting to get back to a 'normal' life after the diagnosis and treatment of breast cancer may find this residue of unexpressed anger to be disabling. It's as if she has nowhere to put it, with no one to listen or maybe no words to express her feelings. She may be afraid of unleashing the fury she holds in her body, or of being seen 'not to cope'. She may even worry about 'boring' her friends and relatives. Anger can signify that we are emotionally hurting, that our needs and wants are not being met or that something isn't right for us. Our anger can also tell us that we are ignoring something which is important to us, that we are giving more than we want to others, or that others are doing too much for us. We are often saying 'no' inside to the 'yes' we are giving out to others.

Betty made an interesting discovery for herself during her counselling sessions at BACUP. She said 'It's as if I have to ask permission of myself to be angry, and that I am worried I will upset others.' When asked what would happen if she upset others, Betty was surprised that she said 'People will disapprove of me, they will think I am ungrateful and they won't like me.' Linking these thoughts to her moment of anger towards her doctor, Betty then realized that she had a wonderful way of silencing herself and blocking out her anger. She often thought 'What's the point of being angry, it won't get me anywhere.' Betty did not believe that she had a right to be angry, or that her anger was legitimate.

It is not wrong to have angry feelings. It is an important part of living and being alive. Anger can be a wonderful, empowering and energizing emotion. Anger mobilizes a lot of energy which seeks to find expression in contact. When this doesn't happen, a cycle is left incomplete and we are left with something which is unfinished. We may be able to divert the energy temporarily, distract ourselves in various ways, become sad, depressed or irritable or very focused on other people. We may busy ourselves and rush back to work to appear efficient, eager to attract admiration for how well we are dealing with our cancer and recovery. But in the end, the original cause of the anger seeks expression, and will find a way out. All our emotions are signals to which we need to pay attention. Anger particularly is a signal which we may be tempted to ignore, and should not.

The experience of having cancer, and the changes that it brings within the body and psyche as well as the family, is different for each individual. But there are certain similarities in the needs of each case; we all need to 'chew over' everything that happens to us in order to assimilate. Just as in the process of eating, when we use oral 'aggression' to break down food into manageable pieces, with a new experience we need to use our aggression in order to understand, to chew over and discard bits which don't feel right. In this way we only swallow and digest those experiences which are acceptable.

Betty decided that she had swallowed the experience of being frightened of dying when she was first told she had cancer. Now she decided that she didn't want this fear lingering inside her. She began to let go of the anger towards her surgeon: 'Even talking about things I haven't spoken about to anyone else has made such a difference. I already feel easier inside. Don't ask me how. I just do and I am beginning to understand more about me.'

Paradoxically, any crisis can offer the opportunity to change our lives, and women have told us that many of the things they had been doing before their cancer no longer felt right. Having breast cancer really brought this into focus. I remember one woman telling me that she had always wanted a dog. Her husband had continuously persuaded her that it wasn't a good idea. On the way home from hospital, she said 'I am buying a dog because I have always wanted one, and still do.' A dog was bought. Importantly, she felt a new sense of energy inside herself, a sense of choice and control of her own life.

The Chinese character for trauma translates as 'opportunity riding on a dangerous wind'. How can this be true of the trauma of cancer? With the diagnosis of a life-threatening illness, the individual gains a new perspective on his or her problems. Many of the rules by which we live can suddenly seem insignificant when faced with our own mortality. In effect what this threat can do is give us permission to act in ways that did not seem possible before. Anger and hostility can now be expressed, assertive behaviour is now allowed. Illness permits the person to say 'no'.

With skilled and experienced support a woman can be encouraged to work through this important stage of her recovery and to uncover a new way of being herself. Cancer brings about so much change. An important change is learning the joy of anger, how to use it positively to give energy, learning to release the stress inside, choosing not to take in new stresses, and recognizing and having a new awareness of what we want and need from life.

18

Reclaiming the sensual self

ANNE HOOPER

I felt as if my husband would never see me as a sexy woman again. I found it difficult to even sleep next to him. Actually he was marvellous and told me repeatedly that he loved and fancied me. But I just couldn't believe him.

Time and again women tell this story after surgery. The details may vary but the ingredients are the same: loss of confidence, a new self-consciousness, inability to talk about feelings of grief, a partner's inability to talk and, occasionally, a depression that won't be shaken off.

Partners, in their turn, with the best of intentions, may not handle the fragile balance of emotions well:

I told her that her scars made no difference to how I felt. But she refused to take it in. The result was she wouldn't make love. We'd get as far as cuddling and stroking, but the minute my hands got anywhere near her breasts she froze.

This husband wasn't able to take on board that just because *he* felt alright didn't guarantee his wife felt the same. Nor did he deduce that if the breasts become a no-go area, then it's wise to work around them, thereby giving his partner time in which to get used to the changes. Further iniquities in this fraught field include: not tuning in to a partner's anxieties, dismissing her anxieties, rushing things, clumsiness, insensitivity, selfishness.

Physical after-effects of breast surgery

Surgery and general anaesthetic are literally depressing. It takes the body systems time to readjust to normal, and during this period everyday life is seen through a fog of depression. This is a physical depression with emotional side-effects. One of these side-effects may well be the depression of libido, with the result that women won't seek lovemaking, nor be able to respond to it.

Emotional after-effects

Women who have lost a breast experience grief. Grief is a depressing emotion, so here is a second layer of depression which again sublimates sexuality. A woman needs time therefore to recover both physically and emotionally. If lovemaking is rushed there can be several unlooked-for outcomes. These may be:

- Women block their feelings and literally anaesthetize their sexuality; they may go through the motions sexually in order to keep the peace, but won't feel anything. A partner may feel upset or guilty in response. Women may feel angry and unloving as a result.
- In the past, a couple may have depended on a pattern of using lovemaking for comfort, for making up after a quarrel, for regaining a sense of security, for feeling safe in a hostile world. When the tried-and-true pattern fails to work in this traumatic circumstance,

each individual feels exposed. What can they do next? Not everyone behaves well when so vulnerable.

- On a personal basis, it is common to go through a loss of confidence about yourself as a woman. Breasts are such a symbol of femininity that, especially when you are naturally depressed, it is hard to believe you will be feminine again. Femininity here equals power, effectiveness, attractiveness, feminine energy and sheer lust.

All in all, it makes a lot of sense to take a rain-check on sex for a while.

Working on yourself

Physical recovery from major surgery is conservatively calculated to take at least two months. If the sufferer has also endured radiotherapy and chemotherapy it will be longer. Ask your medical advisers how long they reckon your body needs to recover physically. Then understand that period is at *least* how long it will take before sexual feelings start seeping back. While you wait for the return of physical wellbeing, put in some work on yourself.

Facing a dangerous illness often has the side-effect of making you radically rethink personal priorities. But, because you are feeling wounded and weak, you may not be able to *do* much to change things at the time. This, in turn, makes you feel frustrated and inferior. People who feel inferior are not good at experiencing and enjoying marvellous sex. Which is why tackling some easy assertion exercises is a good first move.

Assertion exercises are not just about getting what you want. They are (much more importantly) about making yourself feel powerful and effective. By achieving small tasks you feel stronger within. As you feel emotional strength return, you move on to bigger tasks. If your inferiorities are now focused on sexuality, you can make those assertion moves become loving, sensual ones.

Silvia was frightened she wouldn't be able to climax after having surgery. She gave herself three priorities. The first was to say no to her husband when he wanted sex – not something she found easy. The second was to practise a self-massage routine that resulted in self-satisfaction. And the third was to take these new massage techniques into her marriage and practise them with her husband.

Saying no allowed Silvia to feel stronger. She was amazed and thrilled to discover that her husband understood and sympathized. Self-massage and self-stimulation showed her that sensuality actually could and did seep back into her body. She was enormously reassured by this, overcoming her fears. Her success with the second priority allowed her to feel strong enough to take her rediscovered sensuality back into her marriage and to initiate mutual massage. This gave her good sensual contact once more with her partner. Because it felt under her control, her confidence grew once again.

Sexual recovery assertion training programme

- The YES/NO exercise. In one week, say YES to three things that you really want to do and NO to three things that you really don't want to do. This allows you to establish what are your priorities and to act on them. The actions don't have to be sexual ones, and can be either world-shaking or banal. But the exercise is also useful in tackling difficult subjects with your partner concerning sex.
- Self-massage and self-stimulation. Give yourself regular hours of privacy when you can enjoy a warm bath, then self-massage in a warm room. Use warm massage oil and explore your body, noting

which areas feel sensual and which don't. On the first occasion, leave out the genitals. Introduce the genitals on subsequent occasions and gradually pay more attention to the genitals and rather less to the whole body as the weeks go by. If you experience flashes of sensation in the genitals, try to build on these. If you find you are approaching orgasm, feel good about experiencing it.

- Mutual massage. Once you believe you are becoming more sensual in yourself again, share that sensuality with your partner.

Working at the relationship

Partners may have had some obstacles to leapfrog, too. If they are naturally good at expressing themselves there may be no barriers between you. But if they bottle up feelings, you might like to consider the following:

- Offer up some of your own fears about sexuality, then invite theirs.
- Deliberately plan a talking time when nothing else will claim their attention.
- Follow the time-honoured method of asking them about their anxieties for the future while relaxing after an excellent meal.
- Prepare yourself to hear some things that may not be entirely welcome. If you can't cope, don't invite confidences until you feel you can.
- Tell them about other people's reactions so that they feel less isolated and alone.
- If they won't talk, ask them to go to a counsellor with you. BACUP would be very helpful here. BACUP might also be able to help with information about other partner's reactions (*see Directory*).

What do you do when you've got them to unload their anxieties? Understand that confessions are cathartic. Your ability to hear their confession and accept their worries is a major part of the recovery process. If you need help in order to do this, don't hesitate to seek counselling support for yourself.

Exploring sex with your partner

Confessions tend to lead to renewed closeness, so use these moments to move physically closer.

- Cuddle, hug, stroke, use all the warmth moves that come naturally. Let this closeness be the introduction to mutual caresses that are sensual.
- If you're scarred, tell them how much you love being touched but ask them, just for the time being, to avoid certain areas.
- As you feel physically stronger, take the risk of getting more sexual. Use your massage methods on your partner and ask them to do the same to you.
- Once you get comfortable with the intimacy this engenders, the next step, to full lovemaking, isn't so immense.

Sexual enhancement model

If lovemaking *doesn't* come easily, try something based on sex-therapy methods:

- Massage each other's bodies first, with intercourse banned and with genital touching banned.
- Continue the massage, only now include the genitals.
- Focus more fully on the genitals but don't ignore the rest of the body.
- Move on to full lovemaking when *you* feel like it.

These stages can be followed over a period of weeks, and could be timed to tie in with physical recovery and the lifting of both depression and libido. If any of this remains difficult, seek either counselling or sex therapy.

Flash points
What do I do if my partner won't respond at all?
Understand that they need time just as you do. Give them a break for a while, but foster other sorts of closeness and intimacy. Try again a month or so later. If they continue not to respond, suggest you seek counselling. If they refuse to accompany you, go on your own. I can't stress enough how much time is important here as part of the emotional healing process. However, for your own sake it's also important to give yourself a 'time contract'. Work out how long you can reasonably continue in such a difficult situation. If when that period is up, be it one year or even two, things still aren't right, then make yourself your personal priority and decide how you might best move on. I hope it doesn't come to that.

My partner understands I don't want to be rushed. But when we cuddle,
which I really love, he gets aroused and then bad-tempered.
As soon as you have some energy, ask yourself if you could give them some version of lovemaking that doesn't include penetration or strenuous activity on your part. Would oral sex or masturbation be a possibility? It might calm the situation down.

For more information on lovemaking techniques and sexual massage, see
Anne Hooper's Ultimate Sex Guide and *Anne Hooper's Ultimate Sexual Touch*
(Dorling Kindersley).

19

Partners' feelings

John Hobson's wife Judy died on January 9th, 1993. She was 38 and had fought breast cancer for several years. John, 44, a computer professional and Judy, a BBC researcher, met in September 1988 and married in 1991.

When I first met Judy I couldn't believe how well we got on. She was such a cheerful, positive and optimistic person, always smiling. We shared the same bizarre sense of humour. I was overwhelmed really by how good it was, how happy we were. A couple of months after we met Judy and I were talking about the past, and she told me she had had a malignant lump removed from her breast three years previously. The doctors told her after her surgery that she was completely free of breast cancer. I suppose it was unwise of them, because she then felt she was cured.

I remember she said 'It will probably get me in the end'; but she didn't mean it would happen soon, she was sure she was clear. It was a surprise at first but it didn't seriously concern me because she'd been free of it for so long. It certainly didn't enter my mind to say 'I can't cope with this; goodbye.' Our discussion was a fair exchange of problems, if you like. She told me about the breast cancer, and I told her about my previous marriage and my two children.

I knew nothing about breast cancer and what it entailed, I had no reason to. Then, in December 1988 Judy rang me at work to tell me she had found another lump on the scar of the first lump. We were plunged into trauma. The worst aspect is you simply don't know what will happen. The lump could be something or it could be harmless. I thought 'Things were going too well, maybe it's doomed now; I am going to lose this wonderful relationship.' That was my immediate reaction, that I was paying the price for having had something so good.

It comforts me now that she had me to call, that I was there for her, that I was listening and not panicking. Judy's attitude was to tackle things positively, head on. She read all about it and had as much knowledge as possible. That's not my way; I simply focused on her. All the way along she made the choice of what to do next, everything was her decision.

I put on a brave face. I didn't want to put my fears and trauma in front of her. I knew if I explained my worries she would be taking on an extra burden, so I kept them to myself even though I sometimes felt like shrivelling up into a little ball. I was scared of her dying, and I hated seeing what the treatment was doing to her. She in turn was extremely worried it would drive me away.

Judy had the second lump removed, and more radiotherapy. She had a series of hospital appointments to go to, and I always went with her. I was there for the check-up results, and I am sure this made us much closer. We had a common enemy. It compressed time for us; in the back of our mind was the thought we had to make each day special before we found out the next lot of test results.

I didn't cry at any point, even in that last week of her dying, when things were so unbearable. I couldn't cry; I think now that was a mistake. I had the idea I couldn't let the side down. I was conscious of being emotionally vulnerable, but I didn't want her to see it. I just quietly got on with things, although there were times when I panicked and I felt like getting away. I remember I was due to go to the States on business; I felt I needed to go for a break, to get away. But she clearly needed me to stay as she was going into hospital. Now I feel ashamed and guilty that I felt that need to escape at that time. But I am a very independent person and have always got on with my own life; I do need space and it was difficult for me.

We made sure we had the best times together. We went out for lovely meals, looked forward to holidays. We went to Florence, Venice and the States. It was on a trip to California that I had one of the most down moments: we were in a little B & B and it was wonderful, but Judy was so depressed because she was due to go into hospital on our return, and that upset me so much.

Judy retired from the BBC as the cancer began to spread. In April 1991 she was out shopping and her hip snapped. The cancer had become secondary cancer and spread to her bones. She had a hip replacement and her other hip had to be pinned, too. Seeing her after the operation was one of the lowest moments. She wasn't herself at all, she looked so ill and I was terribly upset but I didn't show it. I went home and collapsed emotionally; she never saw that.

It was a bad time for us. She was on morphine and that really makes you a different person; it's hard. Her looks became a concern for her, it was upsetting for her to have a puffy face because of the steroids she had to take. But we had so much to contend with this really wasn't a big deal. Her appearance didn't worry me, it was obvious by then I wasn't going to leave her, she was reassured I would always stick by her. We just got our heads down and got on with life.

The physical side of the relationship caused a lot of worry for Judy too. The effects of her treatment made her tired and the stress of what was happening affected us both physically. Gradually and insidiously the cancer tried to destroy that side of our relationship. In previous relationships she'd felt that when the physical side lapsed it meant the relationship was going wrong. She felt that a bit with us, but it wasn't true at all. She was desperately unhappy about it and fought against it. I reassured her I didn't marry 'Judy with breast cancer', I married 'Judy'.

In the last few months I was a kind of spokesman for us. The family would ring for updates and I took Judy's lead, being as positive as possible. I worked from home, so we were hardly ever apart – Judy in one room, me in another by the phone. It was a pressure sometimes, being that contact point for everyone else. But we had this 'party line' for enquiries, which reflected Judy's optimism. We handled everything together, that is how you have to be. We were fortunate we had Christie hospital in Manchester, who were superb and who so greatly admired Judy's stance of making all the decisions for herself.

On New Year's Eve in 1993 I found her asleep and couldn't wake her up. She went to hospital and stayed there until she died. She was in a coma for a few days, but the moment she was awake she was talking about where we would take our next holiday; she never ever gave up hope. Times when I thought it was impossible, so desperate and awful, she was still positive. 'When can I go home?' she would ask me. Nine days later she died.

It's tough to say what other partners should do in these situations. No amount of knowledge makes it any easier. When your wife dies you become a different person, so now it is difficult to remember how I was then. I try to hold the whole thing in my memory, my time with Judy was such a lovely thing to have had. I think the only thing

Feelings

I regret is that I wish I had done more to make sure I was as loving as possible, loving in a practical way. It got difficult at times to keep that in my mind as practical day-to-day things got in the way.

After she died I found it almost impossible to cope, I don't remember much of it. We did everything as a team, everything was in relation to her, so I was lost on my own. I felt it was my responsibility to deal with the pain by myself. I wrote all my feelings in a diary which I kept every day for a year, and that helped me. I don't think you ever get over something like this. It hits me hard now and again. But I am so glad I met Judy, that we found each other, because it was so right.

Some time after Judy's death I discovered that Dena, a mutual friend, had lost her partner eight years before. She understood what I was going through and it was a tremendous help to me that I could talk to her about my feelings.

I will always love Judy, and at the same time I find I have the strength to look forward to the future. This experience has taught me so much about life.

VIII

Science and Research:
Now and the Future

Many years ago one of my greatest friends was affected by this disease in her twenties. Her strength and courage was an inspiration to all of us, and the devastation felt by her young family and friends was overwhelming. It is essential that more finance is combined with knowledge and research in order that a cure can be found. This initiative enables us all to do something to help find that cure, and I am delighted to offer my support.
Betty Jackson

20

Breast cancer research: tomorrow's world

VIVIENNE PARRY

We live in the age of instant communication. We command, and it is done. So why is it that we cannot get to the bottom of breast cancer, and why is everyone always calling for more research, when so much seems to have been undertaken already? Part of the problem is that, as we have seen, breast cancer has many causes. A range of complex interactions produce what the layperson perceives to be the same end-result. If there is one certainty about breast cancer it is that, although there may be common themes, there will be no universal cure nor any one preventative panacea.

Researching breast cancer is like walking into a field covered in thousands of stones; we are told that pieces of information are hidden under the stones. Some stones will have no information beneath them, but nevertheless they have to be turned over; the act of finding no information is not a setback – simply one less stone that has to be turned over in the future. Other stones will reveal information which seems to have no relevance, until further information comes to light. All the time, information has to be processed, digested and continuously reassessed. Progress in understanding will mostly be fragmented, slow and laborious. Only occasionally will there be a sudden leap forward, as a new piece of information draws a dozen seemingly unconnected facts together to produce an advance that can be shouted from the rooftops. Such an advance can only be possible because of all the previous stone-turning. Such is research. Frustrating, slow, tediously methodical but, without it, there is no rational basis for future treatment, no understanding and no promise for the future.

Read any of the cancer journals and you will discover reams of seemingly incomprehensible hieroglyphics, mostly relating to cancer at a cellular level. Thanks to great leaps in technology, the last few years have seen an explosion of knowledge about cancer at the cellular level and the molecular level. This work is vitally important because it provides information about the steps that turn a normal cell into a malignant one. Only now is that information beginning to be translated into practical help for breast cancer sufferers, and it has taken years of effort and many millions of pounds to get this far.

Current applied research falls broadly into four categories: prevention; screening to identify women at high risk; improved detection; and improved treatment. At present, most lives are likely to be saved by improvements in treatment, because for the foreseeable future women will continue to develop breast cancer. Improved treatments are perhaps the area of research where there is most good news to report.

Risk factors and prevention

There are a large number of known risk factors for breast cancer, which interact in a complex way to initiate and promote the disease. It is said for instance that the most likely woman to have breast cancer is a fat white elderly nun, living in a cold climate in the western hemisphere, with a high dietary fat intake, who started her periods early and whose mother and sisters had breast cancer. The most potent risk factor – increasing age – is one that we can do nothing to alter. Neither can we alter our genes (of which more later). Much research is concentrated on the preventative effects of diet – particularly vitamin A intake and a low-fat diet. The largest study on diet and cancer (the European Prospective Investigation into Cancer, or EPIC) is currently being undertaken. Breast cancer results are expected in about five years' time. It has been claimed that deaths from breast cancer might be cut in half by changes to women's diets. However, smaller trials have failed to show conclusive evidence that this is the case. Even if diet were shown to be of such great importance, I believe it is still unlikely that women would change their dietary habits to the extent that might be required; a Japanese diet containing about 20 per cent fat would seem very austere to a westerner. The depressing failure of health messages about high-fat diets and the increased risk of heart attack shows that dietary manipulation is hard to achieve.

Hormonal status is another risk factor; in effect, the longer the breasts are exposed to circulating reproductive hormones, principally oestrogen, the more likely a woman is to have breast cancer. Three key events – age at first period, age at first pregnancy and age at menopause – play their part in determining risk. As we have seen, one of the reasons why western women have more breast cancers may be because they have more ovulations in their lifetime; women who have their ovaries surgically removed are known to be at greatly reduced risk.

There are therefore two possible preventative strategies by pharmaceutical means: to prevent the production of the potent oestrogen derivative; and to muzzle the ovaries, so preventing them producing reproductive hormones. There are some promising drugs called gonadotrophin releasing hormone agonists (GnRHAs) which might do the latter, but the incidence of side-effects would make them unacceptable to well women. In any case, women are suspicious of long-term drug therapy. For this reason, the other potential drug preventative agent – tamoxifen – may also fail. At present tamoxifen is used as a successful adjuvant therapy, which means it is given to women with breast cancer at the time of treatment; it is credited with a 30 per cent increase in survival rates. Tamoxifen is an anti-hormone agent – very similar to many oral contraceptives – and rather than just give it to women who already have breast cancer, it has been suggested that it should be given to well women at high risk, in whom it might produce a reduction in breast cancer of about one third. There is a large trial of tamoxifen under way at the moment, but it is beset with difficulties, not least of which is the State of California declaring tamoxifen to be carcinogenic; its future seems less rosy than it once was. Despite the controversy, it may be that the possible benefits outweigh the risks, but further research is required before this can be established conclusively.

Future research on prevention will also target the influence of environmental contaminants which mimic oestrogens – called xenoestrogens – as they might play a role in the increasing incidence of breast cancer. A bewildering variety of everyday chemicals are involved, and even if they can be identified, they are so common in everyday life that they will be hard to avoid.

You may be wondering where a possible breast cancer vaccine fits into the prevention picture. While to the public a vaccine is a preventative measure, to cancer scientists a cancer vaccine is a way of mobilizing the body's immune system to fight an already diagnosed cancer. Combined with early detection, cancer vaccines are promising, but a very, very long way down the road. A cancer vaccine in the prophylactic sense is the stuff of science fiction – so don't hold your breath on this one.

The final plank in the prevention research strategy relates to stress. In December 1995, the *British Medical Journal* published the results of a study showing breast cancer to be more prevalent in those who had high levels of stress in their lives – such as bereavement, divorce and so on. This study puts into scientific black and white what many have always suspected, and makes it more likely that stress-reduction techniques will be the subject of future scientific research related to cancer prevention.

Screening and detection

Improved screening leading to earlier treatment is perhaps the most exciting area of research. By the time a woman is able to feel a lump of about 1 centimetre in diameter in her breast, about 100 million cells are involved. It all starts with one rogue cell, and each cell takes 48 hours to double, so a 1-centimetre lump may have been a cancer for as long as six or eight years. The concept of a molecular mammogram has been floated; essentially rather than pick up cancers at an advanced stage, a molecular mammogram would, by identifying changes in genetic code, pinpoint a cancer at the very earliest stage, when treatment might be most successful.

In cancer, changes in the genetic make-up of a cell – called mutations – occurring at some time during life rather than at birth, are usually the problem. The example most familiar to us is exposure to radiation. Every time a cell divides, genetic information has to be faithfully copied and reproduced. The more active the tissue (and breast tissue is constantly on the go – just note the change in size produced by your monthly cycle), the more cell divisions there are. The more cell divisions, the greater the chance of there being a copying error. This explains why the risk of cancer increases as you get older – there has simply been more opportunity for copying errors to have been made. When there are genetic errors in cells, their offspring seem to lose the ability to divide and multiply in a controlled way. It now appears that some cancers – including breast cancer – result from an interaction between an inherited genetic dictate (which by itself is incapable of producing a cancerous transformation) and a second genetic error, at the cellular level, which somehow allows the malignant intention of the inherited gene to be translated into reality.

Although there have been exciting advances in discovering the genes causing familial breast cancer (see Dr Miriam Stoppard's piece, *page 24*), the realization of new drugs based on these findings will take at least a decade. In the short term, research is urgently needed to produce improved, more accurate breast imaging for diagnosis. Mammograms currently use a 40-year-old technology to find small lumps in women's breasts. But advances are coming; for instance software which was originally used for computer vision by the military is now being used to scan mammograms with far greater accuracy. Other imaging techniques such as magnetic resonance imaging (MRI scanning) may be used in the future to screen women who are known to be at particularly high risk, or perhaps younger women whose denser breast tissue makes conventional imaging problematic. Future alternatives to imaging may exploit the fact that there is a tiny difference in electric current between the interior and exterior of a cell which may be disrupted in cancerous cells. A breast biofield examination, currently under trial, can detect such changes through a special sensor placed on the skin. Such examinations can avoid unnecessary biopsies for benign conditions.

Treatment

Treatment is where advances are really paying dividends. Survival rates are increasing all the time. Genetic changes in cells are known to be hugely important in the control of cancer. The possibility that gene therapy – introducing correct copies of genes directly into tumours – might be of benefit is a fine theory which has excited great attention. In practice it has proved immensely difficult to introduce correct gene copies in large enough amounts to be effective. Until a better gene-delivery system is perfected, gene therapy will remain a treatment of future potential only. However, it is immensely important that basic research, which will allow scientists to understand how to improve such gene-delivery systems, continues.

Some breast cancers are more aggressive than others. Early recognition of this fact allows appropriate treatment. For instance, some breast cancers have lost receptors for the hormones oestrogen and progesterone. You might think that this would make them less likely to grow. Not a bit of it. These are the mean dudes of the breast cancer world – resistant to drug treatments such as tamoxifen – and aggressive and dangerous to boot. The discovery that these changes are linked to mutations in a particular gene pinpoints a future role for gene therapy in this type of cancer. Identifying the protein products of breast cancers can also point to a therapy, because there is an increased likelihood that a drug therapy which disrupts the production of the protein will have anti-cancer activity.

Chemotherapy has greatly improved, but one of the side-effects of cytotoxic drugs is that they knock out white blood cells, the very cells trying to fight off the cancer, as well as the cancer itself. Giving substances called cytokines, in particular one which stimulates white cells called granulocyte colony stimulating factor (GCSF), makes women having chemotherapy feel better. It may also allow larger, more effective doses of chemotherapy to be given. Another treatment with a similar rationale is autologous bone marrow transplantation, which involves taking a sample of a woman's own bone marrow before high-dose chemotherapy is started, and storing it until it can be safely replaced after the chemotherapy course has been completed.

Research has led to the development of a number of new drugs for the treatment of advanced breast cancer. Of particular promise are drugs which suppress oestrogen called aromatase inhibitors. These drugs stop production of oestrogen completely, so preventing cancer cells from growing. Tumours require a constant blood supply if they are to continue growing, and a great deal of research is currently aimed at finding ways to disrupt the blood supply to tumours (so-called anti-angiogenesis). There are drugs currently on trial which may interfere with angiogenesis, so walling in the tumour and preventing spread. Although applicable to all solid tumours, these drugs may be of particular use in breast cancer.

The research I have outlined above does not include advances in surgery, breast conservation, new ways of delivering radiotherapy using implants, or the use of lasers in treatment. Nor does it include the advances in understanding the psychological help required to maximize women's ability to cope with breast cancer. All of these current treatments have been subject to clinical trials and have arisen as a result of extensive research by many types of scientists and doctors, funded mainly by charities.

Contrary to public opinion, there is very little central government funding for basic cancer research. Without research, there can be no advances in treatment. Without public money, research cannot continue. And in research lies our hope for the future.

Afterword

DR BARRY GUSTERSON

There is no doubt that improvements in surgery, chemotherapy, hormone therapy and, more recently, the breast screening programme, will all continue to make important contributions towards saving the lives of thousands of women each year in the United Kingdom. Whilst these important advances have been taking place in the management of breast cancer, there has been a revolution taking place in medical sciences.

New technology is now assisting in the rapid identification of the genetic abnormalities that convert a normal cell into a cancer cell. In the last two years this has resulted in the identification of four genes responsible for familial breast cancer, and there are now more than twenty other genes thought to cause the growth of breast cancers and their spread. All of these genes are possible new targets for drug design. It is predicted that in the next ten years the majority, if not all, of the genes that cause breast cancer will be known. We have to be careful, however, to keep the balance between the excitement and hope that these new findings bring, and the realism that finding a gene is only the beginning. It takes many years to go from the gene to new treatments, with many false starts along the way.

To ensure that these findings are harnessed as quickly as possible for the benefit of present patients as well as the women of tomorrow, we have to bring together experts in different branches of science. They can then combine their knowledge and expertise to work out the functions of the genes that cause breast cancer. This is the logical way forward, and this is why we need a dedicated Breast Cancer Centre. It is also important that the work in the centre is complementary to, and integrated with, that being supported by the other major charities, government, industry and other scientists around the world.

As our knowledge of the complexity of breast cancer grows, it is clear that we are unlikely to have a single cure, or a single breakthrough. Producing a multidisciplinary and stimulating scientific environment devoted to breast cancer will, however, ensure that the individual 'Breakthroughs' come as soon as possible, and that they will be directed to the benefit of all.

Professor B A Gusterson Ph.D., F.R.C.Path., Professor of Histopathology and Chairman of the Section of Cell Biology and Experimental Pathology at the Institute of Cancer Research. Consultant at the Royal Marsden Hospital. Sutton, February 1996

IX

Useful Information

Glossary

Adjuvant Treatment

Treatment given in addition to the primary treatment.

AIDS and Breast Cancer

Women with AIDS do not appear to have a higher breast cancer risk than the average woman.

Antioxidant

Vitamins A, C and E are examples of a group of chemicals which will combine with toxic substances (called free radicals) in the body to make them harmless.

Atypical Hyperplasia

This describes an increase of cells in the lining of the ducts and lobules in the breast. These cells are abnormal, but not cancer.

Axilla

The underarm.

Axillary Nodes

Doctors may feel under your arm to check for enlarged glands (lymph nodes). Not a very helpful check, as it is not an accurate indicator of whether breast cancer is present.

Benign
Non-cancerous.

Bilateral Mastectomy
Surgical removal of both breasts.

Biopsy
Taking a sample of breast tissue to examine under a microscope for signs of cancerous cells. Less often used than fine needle aspiration cytology.

BRCA1
This is a gene that is abnormal in 5 per cent of patients with breast cancer, and is responsible for approximately half of all cases of familial breast cancer.

BRCA2
This was the second breast cancer gene identified that has a role in familial breast cancer. This exciting advance was made by a research team led by Dr Mike Stratton at the Institute of Cancer Research in London, and was the major achievement in the fight against breast cancer in 1995.

Breast Awareness
Knowing what is normal for your body. See a doctor if there are any changes in the appearance or feel of your breasts.

Breast Cancer
Cancer occurs when the cells lining the ends of the units that make up the breast (lobules) start to multiply out of normal control. These cells form a lump.

Carcinogen
Any substance that, when exposed to living tissue, may cause the production of cancer.

Chemotherapy
Cancer-killing drugs which are given to mop up cancer cells that have spread outside the breast, or to shrink a lump prior to surgery. It is usually offered to women with large lumps, axillary lymph nodes which contain cancerous cells, or disease elsewhere in the

body (metastases). Side-effects are common and debilitating, but the aim is to improve one's chances of survival.

Cyclical Mastalgia

Breast pain, worse just before periods.

Cysts

Harmless and common. This is a swollen duct or lobule containing fluid. Can usually be diagnosed with ultra-sound scan. Fine needle aspiration confirms that there is no cancer and usually makes the cyst disappear.

Discharge from Nipple

Nipple discharge is common and usually harmless. If it is blood-stained, persistent and troublesome, it should be investigated with examination, mammogram and biopsy if there is any worry about underlying cancer.

Dissemination

Cancer cells spreading via the blood or lymphatic fluid.

Ductal Carcinoma In Situ (DCIS)

A type of cancer involving the breast ducts, the tubes which conduct milk from the milk-forming parts of the breast to the nipple. 'In situ' means the cancer only involves the ducts.

Duct Ectasia

This common condition in elderly women causes nipple discharge, often on one breast only. It is harmless.

Eczema Nipple

Eczema or red skin on the breast may be part of a more generalized eczema which causes dry and itchy skin. A single patch of eczema overlying a nipple needs to be investigated to ensure there is no underlying cancer.

Endogenous

Arising within the body.

Epidemiology

The study of disease within populations, and its relationship to environmental, social and hereditary factors.

Evening Primrose Oil

A useful treatment for breast pain which is worse just before periods (cyclical mastalgia).

Excision Biopsy

An operation to remove a breast lump and examine it under the microscope.

Family History

Having a sister, mother or daughter with breast cancer before the age of fifty approximately doubles a woman's risk of developing breast cancer herself. This does not mean that you have an inherited cancer gene in your family, as both you and your relative could have developed a cancer by chance. About 10 per cent of cancers in the west are due to an inherited gene.

Fibroblasts

These lie among the fat and connective tissue of the breast, producing a number of chemical messengers called growth factors. These growth factors seem to communicate with breast cancer cells, possibly stimulating their growth and their ability to spread.

Fine Needle Aspiration Cytology

A fine needle is inserted into a breast lump. Cells are drawn into a syringe and sent to be examined under a microscope. This is an accurate way of telling whether a lump is cancerous or not. It is done with local anaesthetic only.

Hereditary

Transmitted from parents to offspring.

Holistic

The consideration of the whole person in the treatment of disease.

Useful Information

Hormone Replacement Therapy (HRT)
Hormone treatment given to replace levels of oestrogen in women during or after the menopause.

Hormone Therapy
Breast cancers are examined to see whether they have hormone receptors, which means they are more likely to be sensitive to hormonal influences.

Hyperplasia
Increase in the number of normal cells lining the ducts and lobules in the breast (*see* Atypical Hyperplasia).

Lactation (Breastfeeding)
The secretion of milk by the mammary glands of the breast. This process is controlled by hormones. Breastfeeding provides an excellent source of nutrition and protection from infection for a newborn baby, and reduces the risk of breast cancer in the mother. Breastfeeding can cause cracked nipples, inflammation of the breast (mastitis) and infection (abscess). Good advice and help with breastfeeding can help to minimize these problems.

Lipoma
A harmless cause of lumps in the breast. It is a collection of fat cells and can be removed if troublesome or diagnosis uncertain.

Lumpectomy
The surgical removal of a breast lump.

Lymphatic system
A network of thin-walled vessels which drain fluid, known as lymph, from the spaces between cells. The vessels are interrupted by lymph nodes which filter off bacteria and other foreign particles.

Lymphoedema
After surgery and radiotherapy, arms and hands may swell. Women who have had their axillary lymph nodes removed are particularly susceptible.

Male Breast Cancer

Only accounts for 0.5 per cent of all breast cancer, but tends to be fairly advanced by the time it is diagnosed.

Mammogram

An X-ray of the breast.

Mammography

A process in which the breast is squashed between two plates and X-rays passed through to give a picture of the breast tissue (mammogram).

Mastectomy

Operation to remove a breast. It removes breast tissue with some overlying skin, and usually the nipple. Breast reconstruction can be done at the same time.

Metastases

Spread of cancer cells to other parts of the body. Breast cancer cells may spread in the bloodstream to lungs, bones, liver, brain, and may also spread to the opposite breast.

MRI (Magnetic Resonance Imaging)

A method to produce a three-dimensional picture of a tumour in the body using a safe form of radiation and a large magnet.

Oestrogen

One of the group of steroid hormones that control female sexual development, promoting the growth and function of the female sex organs and female secondary sexual characteristics such as breast development.

Oncology

The branch of medicine that deals with the treatment of cancer.

Oophorectomy

Removal of the ovaries.

Useful Information

Ovarian Suppression
A treatment for breast cancer which stops the ovaries producing oestrogen. Done by giving a low dose of radiation to the ovaries, or by surgical removal of the ovaries.

Paget's Disease
An eczema-like condition overlying the nipple. It can indicate underlying cancer in the breast.

Pain in Breast
Very common. Hardly ever a sign of cancer.

Pathologist
Medical specialist who interprets results of biopsies.

Pathology
The branch of medicine concerned with the cause, origin and nature of disease.

PET (Positron Emission Tomography)
A method of following chemicals in the body that are labelled with radioactive isotopes. This is used to see tumours in the body and to follow the distribution of drugs.

Prophylactic Mastectomy
An operation to remove the breast as a measure to prevent the occurrence of cancer.

Prosthesis
A physical substitute for a part of the body, for example a breast form used to fill out a bra after mastectomy.

Quadrantectomy
Breast conservation surgery is the alternative to mastectomy. It involves removal of the tumour (lump) with surrounding normal tissue (wide local excision or lumpectomy), or a more extensive removal of the quarter of the breast in which the lump is located.

Radiotherapist/Radiographer
A medical expert in radiotherapy.

Radiotherapy
The use of radiation to target and kill cancer cells.

Radiotherapy Action Group Exposure (RAGE)
A group calling for government compensation on behalf of women who have suffered severe nerve damage as a result of radiotherapy treatments.

Reconstruction
Cosmetic operation to reconstitute a normal breast shape, which can be carried out at the time of removal of the breast tissue, or later.

Secondaries
Cancers which have spread into the rest of the body from cells travelling from the primary, or original, tumour.

Segmentectomy (Wedge)
The removal of the segment of the breast containing cancer.

Staging
A way of assessing the extent of disease when breast cancer is diagnosed. Factors taken into account are size of tumour, involvement of lymph nodes (glands), and presence of any metastases. Treatment options can then be assessed and an indication given as to the outlook.

Subcutaneous Mastectomy
An operation where breast tissue is removed from beneath the skin and an implant inserted, leaving the nipple and areola intact.

Tamoxifen
A synthetic hormonal drug used in cancer treatment and prevention.

Tumour
A growth; can be benign (harmless) or malignant (cancerous).

Useful Information

Ultra-sound

Harmless sound waves used to gain an image of breast lumps, often in younger women who have dense breasts so that mammography is less useful. Very good at showing up cysts.

Virginal Hypertrophy

Normal breast development that occurs around puberty; may be asymmetrical and can sometimes cause abnormally large breasts in adolescent girls, which may cause embarrassment and discomfort. There is no increased risk of cancer.

Special thanks to Dr Anne Robinson for many of these definitions, and also to Professor Barry Gusterson, Dr Cathy Read and Dr Miriam Stoppard.

Directory

Action Organizations

BREAKTHROUGH Breast Cancer
Tel. 0171–430 2086
Launched in 1991 to raise £15 million to establish the Breast Cancer Research Centre, which will bring together some of the world's best scientists under one roof in a co-ordinated programme of research focused exclusively on this one disease.

The National Cancer Alliance
PO Box 579
Oxford OX4 1LP
Tel. 01865 793 566
A voluntary organization of patients and health care professionals formed to voice concerns and opinions about the services, care and treatment provided for people with cancer. Information about good care and services, standards of care, and in general the treatment people have the right to expect and how to get it. Also supplies *The Directory of Cancer Specialists*, which includes surgeons, oncologists and cancer nurses who specialize in breast cancer.

Radiotherapy Action Group Exposure (RAGE)
Tel. 0181– 460 7476 (breast cancer issues)
Tel. 0161– 839 2927 (all types of cancer)
A support and campaigning group calling for government compensation and better care on behalf of women who have suffered severe damage as a result of radiotherapy treatments.

UK Breast Cancer Coalition
PO Box 8554
London SW8 2ZB
Tel. 0171–720 0945
Fax 0171–978 1632
Launched in July 1995 by broadcaster Nancy Roberts. Its three main aims are: Access, Research, Influence. Membership is open to all. Dedicated to making the voice of women heard in all places where it matters – government, parliament, health authorities, hospitals, doctor's surgeries, research committees, and so on. For more information write enclosing SAE.

UK Breast Cancer Internet Site
http://doric.bart.ucl.ac.uk/web/BreastCancer/aware.html
Breast cancer information, contact numbers, charity campaigns and a list of other cancer-related sites. Contact Marie Nally or Nina Pope, e-mail no. ucftnan ucl.ac.uk

The Women's Environmental Network Trust
Aberdeen Studios
22 Highbury Grove
London N5 2BR
Tel. 0171–354 8823
Addresses environmental issues that specifically affect women. For membership details, or to make a donation, write to the above address. For the *Women's Environmental Network Directory of Information* (WENDI), providing updated information on key consumer issues, call 0171–704 6800.

Women's National Cancer Control Campaign
Suna House
128/130 Curtain Road
London EC2 3AR
Admin: 0171–729 4688
Fax 0171– 613 0771
Helpline: 0171–729 2229
Supports and encourages the provision of facilities for early diagnosis of cancer in women.

Counselling and Practical Advice

BACUP (British Association of Cancer United Patients)
3 Bath Place
Rivington Street
London EC2A 3JR
Admin: 0171–696 9003
Fax 0171–696 9002
BACUP Cancer Information Service 0171–613 2121
Counselling Service: London 0171–696 9000; Glasgow 0141–553 1553
A national charity offering free information and counselling to people with cancer, their families and friends, by telephone or letter. BACUP publishes 46 free booklets on a range of cancers, treatments and practical issues. If you would like to receive a specific booklet please send a large SAE stating which booklet you would like to receive. Also produce a booklet on *Cancer and Complementary Therapies* covering counselling, relaxation, visualization, self-help groups, spiritual healing, meditation, massage, aromatherapy, acupuncture and nutrition.

Useful Information

Breast Cancer Care
Kiln House
210 New Kings Road
London SW6 4NZ
Admin: 0171–384 2984
Fax 0171–384 3387
Helplines:
London 0171–384 2344
Glasgow 0141–353 1050
Edinburgh 0131–221 0407
Nationwide Freeline 0500 245 345

The British Association for Counselling (BAC)
1 Regent Place
Rugby CV21 2PJ
Tel. 01788 550 899
Will supply you with names and addresses of counsellors in your locality. Send SAE
with your request.

The British Association of Sexual and Marital Therapists (BASMT)
PO Box 62
Sheffield S10 3TL
Will supply you with names and address of sex therapists in your locality. Send SAE
with your request.

Cancer Care Society
21 Zetland Road
Redland
Bristol BS6 7AL
Tel: 0117 942 7419
Provides social and emotional support for people with cancer and their families and
friends through a national network of branches. Telephone and personal counselling by

trained counsellors. Offers a link service for people with cancer to be put in touch with one another.

Cancerkin
Royal Free Hospital Breast Cancer Appeal
Pond Street
London NW3 2QG
Tel. 0171–830 2323
Provides advice, support and care for patients with breast cancer and support to those close to them. Also informs, educates and trains health professionals and carers. Provides factual information to the general public. Cancerkin also has a free lymphoedema clinic.

CancerLink
17 Britannia Street
London WC1X 9JN
Admin: 0171–833 2818
Fax 0171–833 4963

9 Castle Terrace
Edinburgh EH1 2DP
Admin: 0131–228 5567
Fax 0131–228 8956
Helplines:
General: 0171–933 2451
Asian Language Line (Hindi & Bengali): 0171–713 7867
For young people affected by cancer: Freephone 0800 591 028
Scotland: 0131–228 5557
Provides emotional support and information in response to telephone enquiries and letters on all aspects of cancer, from people with cancer, their families, friends and professionals working with them. It is a resource to over 500 cancer support and self-help groups throughout Britain, and helps people who set up new groups. Free publications and audio tapes in seven languages also available.

Useful Information

Institute of Family Therapy
43 New Cavendish Street
London W1M 7RG
Tel. 0171–935 1651
The Institute's Elizabeth Raven Memorial Fund offers free counselling to families who have suffered a bereavement within the past twelve months, or those who have seriously ill family members. They work with the whole family and the service is free, but voluntary donations are accepted to help other families.

Support and Care

Cancer Relief Macmillan Fund
Anchor House
15/19 Britten Street
London SW3 3TZ
Helpline: 0171–335 7811
Fax 0171–376 8098
Supports and develops services to provide specialist care for people with cancer at every stage of their illness: Macmillan nurses; Macmillan doctors; Macmillan cancer care and information units. Services usually part of the NHS. Information on Macmillan services on request. Application for patient grants though community, hospital, hospice nurses, social workers and other health care professionals.

Carers' National Association Head Office
20–25 Glasshouse Yard
London EC1A 4JS
Admin: 0171–490 8818
Advice & Information: 0171–490 8898
Offers information and support to people caring for relatives and friends. The Association has over 100 branches all over the UK which are run by carers and can refer carers

to local sources of help and support. Association also has offices in Northern Ireland, Scotland and Wales. Lobbies government, both local and national, on behalf of carers. Offers a range of free leaflets and information sheets.

The Compassionate Friend
53 North Street
Bristol BS3 1EN
Tel. 0117–953 9639
A self-help group of parents whose son or daughter (of any age, including adults) has died from any cause. Quarterly newsletter, postal library, range of leaflets. Personal and group support. Befriending, rather than counselling.

Cruse Bereavement Care
126 Sheen Road
Richmond TW9 1UR
Tel. 0181–940 4818
Helpline: 0181–332 7227 (Mon–Fri 9.30 a.m.–5 p.m.)
Offers free help to all bereaved people through its 194 local branches, by providing both individual and group counselling, opportunities for social contact and practical advice. A list of related publications and a newsletter are available.

Hospice Information Service
St Christopher's Hospice
51–59 Lawrie Park Road
Sydenham
London SE26 6DZ
Publishes a directory of hospice and palliative care services which provides details of hospices, home care teams and hospital support teams in the UK and the Republic of Ireland. For a copy of the directory or details on local services, send SAE and two first-class stamps.

Useful Information

The Imperial Cancer Research Fund (ICRF)
PO Box 123
Lincoln's Inn Fields
London WC2A 3PX
Tel. 0171–242 0200
Will provide a range of leaflets and brochures free if you send SAE.

Marie Curie Cancer Care
28 Belgrave Square
London SW1X 8QG
Tel. 0171–235 3325
Fax 0171–235 2297
Hands-on nursing care is provided day and night by approximately 5,000 Marie Curie nurses in patients' homes throughout the UK. The service is accessed through the local district nursing service. They also run eleven Marie Curie Centres (hospices); admission is by referral by GP or consultant. Both these services are free to cancer patients.

The Sue Ryder Foundation
Cavendish
Sudbury
Suffolk CO10 8AY
Tel. 0178 280 252
There are nine Sue Ryder Homes in England which specialize in cancer care. Visiting nurses also care for patients in their own homes. Advice and bereavement counselling and respite care. For any medical questions, telephone Miss Pam Jowett, Nurse adviser, on 0114 283 0596.

Northern Ireland

Action Cancer
Action Cancer House
1 Marlborough Park
Belfast BT9 6HQ
Tel. 01232 661 081
Has a full-time clinic and mobile unit for breast and cervical screening. Also one-to-one counselling for people and their families, for all types of cancer.

Ulster Cancer Foundation
40–42 Eglantine Avenue
Belfast BT9 6DX
Admin: 01232 663 281
Fax 01232 660 081
Helpline: 01232 663 439
Helplines and information services, including breast care and mastectomy support.

Scotland

Tak Tent Cancer Support Scotland
The Western Infirmary
Block, 20 Western Court
100 University Place
Glasgow G12 6SQ
Admin: 0141–211 1930
Resource Centre: 0141–211 1932
Offers information, support, education and care for cancer patients, families, friends and health professionals. Network of support groups across Scotland.

Useful Information

Wales

Tenovus Cancer Information Centre
PO Box 88, College Buildings
Courtenay Road
Cardiff CF1 1FA
Tel. 01222 497 7000
Fax 01222 489 919
Helpline: 0800 526 527
Publishes a free directory of breast cancer groups and breast cancer nurses in Wales, and supports people with all forms of cancer.

Eire

Irish Cancer Society
5 Northumberland Road
Dublin
Admin: 1 668 1855
Fax 1 668 7599
Helpline: 800 200 700
A national charity working to save lives from breast cancer and improve quality of life for women with breast cancer through research, specialist nursing care, breast awareness programmes and 'Reach and Recovery' support groups.

Holistic and Complementary Medicine

Aromatherapy Organisations Council
3, Latyment Close
Braybrook
Market Harborough
Leics LE16 8LN
Tel. 01858 434242
Send an A5 SAE for an information booklet on aromatherapy and advice on how to find an aromatherapist in your area.

Aromatherapy Trade Council
PO Box 52
Market Harborough
Leics LE16 8ZX
Advice on manufacturers of pure essential oils – aromatherapy oils are not licensed and should not be sold with labels claiming medical benefits. Send SAE for information.

Bach Flower Center
Tel. 01491 834 678
For general enquiries, education, practitioners, and so on. Mail-order only: tel. 0171–495 2404.

The Bristol Cancer Help Centre
Grove House
Cornwallis Grove
Clifton
Bristol BS8 4PG
Seeks to combine the benefits of a holistic approach with an appreciation of the effectiveness of orthodox treatment or surgery.

Useful Information

The Cancer Support Centre Wandsworth
PO Box 17
20–22 York Road
London SW11 3QE
Admin and Helpline: 0171–924 3924
Fax 0171–978 6505
A registered charity working with people with cancer, their families, friends and health professionals. It has a holistic approach and offers information and support, a range of complementary therapies including massage, and offers home-visiting schemes.

The Healing Herbs of Dr Bach
Tel. 01873 890 218
A workshop which will send preparations anywhere in the world.

The Institute of Complementary Medicine
PO Box 194
London SE16
Will supply names of reliable holistic practitioners for treatments such as homoeopathy, relaxation techniques, and osteopathy. Also have contact with various support groups. Please send SAE and two first-class stamps, stating area of interest.

National Institute of Medical Herbalists
Tel. 01392 426 022
Will help you find a herbal practitioner in your area.

Neal's Yard Agency
14 Neal's Yard
London WC2H 9DP
Tel. 0171–379 0141
Free advice on workshops, holidays and courses. Will also help you find a counsellor or psychotherapist. Neal's Yard Remedies, stockist of natural remedies, is at 15 Neal's Yard, London WC2, tel. 0171–379 7222 (mail-order service available, tel. 01865 245 436).

The Research Council for Complementary Medicine
60 Great Ormond Street
London WC1N 3JF
Tel. 0171–833 8897

Society of Homoeopaths
Tel. 01604 21400
Will help you find a qualified homoeopath in your area.

Prostheses

Information

Breast Cancer Care
See page 193 for address

Mail-Order Companies

Amoena (UK) Ltd
14/15 Monks Brook Park
School Close
Chandlers Ford
Hants SO5 3RA
Tel. 0800 378 668

Anita International Ltd
15/16a Eton Garages
Eton Avenue
London NW3 4PE
Tel. 0171–435 2258

Useful Information

Medimac
15/16 St Mary's House
St Mary's Road
Shoreham by Sea
West Sussex BN43 5ZA
Tel. 01273 441 436

Nicola Jane
Lagness
Chichester
West Sussex PO20 6LW
Tel. 01234 268 686

Tru-Life Ltd
9–15 Grundy Street
Liverpool L5 9YH
Tel. 0151–207 5690

Corsetry Specialists

Rigby and Peller
2 Hans Road
London SW13 1RX
Tel. 0171–589 9293
Offers advice to women who need larger bras or have special requirements, for example after mastectomy.

Breast Reconstruction

The British Association of Aesthetic Surgeons
The Royal College of Surgeons
35 Lincoln's Inn Fields
London WC2A 3PA
Tel. 0171–831 5161
For a list of plastic surgeons.

Breastfeeding

La Leche League
Tel. 0171–242 1278
Information and help for women who want to know more about breastfeeding.

Additional Therapies

The British Association of Art Therapists
11a Richmond Road
Brighton
East Sussex BN2 3RL
Tel. 01734 265 407
To find a registered art therapist in your area.

The British Wheel of Yoga
Tel. 01529 306 851
For a yoga or meditation teacher in your area.

Useful Information

Council for Nutrition Education and Therapy
34 Wadham Road
London SW15 2LR
Send cheque or postal order (£2) for the *Nationwide Directory of Nutritionists*. For a free information pack on optimum nutrition, send SAE to Institute for Optimum Nutrition, Blades Court, Deodar Rd, London SW15 2NU.

Gerson Research Organisation
108 Birmingham Road
Litchfield
Staffs WS14 9BW
For information about Gerson nutritional therapy send an A5 SAE.

Society for the Promotion of Nutritional Therapy
PO Box 47
Heathfield
East Sussex TN21 8ZX
Will help you find a nutritional therapist in your area. Send £1 with your request.

Westminster Pastoral Foundation
Tel. 0171–937 6956
Will help you find a psychotherapist.

Women's Nutritional Advisory Service
Tel. 01273 487 366 (general enquiries)
Helplines:
Overcoming PMS Naturally: 0839 556 600
Overcoming the Menopause Naturally: 0839 556 602
For a full list of numbers: 0839 556 615
Information, advice on self-help books; runs clinics, postal and telephone consultations. Will also advise about beating menopausal symptoms without HRT or coming off HRT safely.

Further Reading

'Alcohol Consumption and Mortality Among Women' C. S. Fuchs, M. J. Stampfer, G. A. Colditz, E. L. Giovannucci, J. E. Manson, I. Kawachi, D. J. Hunter, J. E. Hankinson, C. H. Hennekens, B. Rosner *et al.* (Schanning Laboratory, Boston MA), *New England Journal of Medicine* 332 (19), May 11 1995: 1245–50.

Always a Woman: A practical guide to living with breast cancer surgery Carolyn Faulder (Thorsons, 1992).

'Annual Report of the Working Party on Pesticide Residues 1994' (HMSO, 1995; figures taken from 'Chemical Cuisine', *Living Earth*, Autumn 1995, published by The Soil Association).

'Antioxidant Micronutrients and Breast Cancer' M. Garland, W. C. Willet, J. E. Manson, D. J. Hunter (Department of Epidemiology, Harvard School of Public Health, Boston MA), *Journal of American College of Nutrition* 12 (4), August 1993: 400–11.

'Antioxidant Vitamins and Cancer: The Physician's Health Study and Women's Health Study' Julie E. Buring, Charles H. Hennekens (Brigham and Women's Hospital at Harvard Medical School), presentation at the Vitamin E Symposium, Hawaii, June 1995.

Breast Awareness Cathy Cirket (Thorsons, 1992).

The Breast Book: The essential guide to breast care & breast health for all ages Dr Miriam Stoppard (Dorling Kindersley, 1996).

Breast Cancer and Breast Care Carolyn Faulder (Ward Lock, 1995).

'Breast Cancer: Cause and Prevention' Barbara S. Hulka, Azadeh T. Stark, *The Lancet* 346, 30 September 1995.

The Breast Cancer Companion Cathy LaTour (Morrow, 1993).

Breast Care Baum *et al.* (Oxford University Press, 1994).

Breast Is Best Drs Penny and Andrew Stanway (Macmillan, 1996).

Breast Reconstruction Royal Marsden Patient Information Series (available from Haigh & Hochland Publications Ltd, 174a Ashley Road, Hale, Cheshire).

Cancer Information at Your Fingertips V. Speechley and M. Rosenfield (2nd edition, Class Publishing, 1996).

'Carcinogens in Israeli Milk: A Study in Regulatory Failure' J. B. Westin, *International Journal of Health Services* 23 (3), 1993: 497–517.

'Dietary Fat, Calories and the Risk of Breast Cancer in Post-menopausal Women: a prospective population-based study' E. Barrett-Connor, N. J. Friedlander (Department of Family and Preventive Medicine, University of California), *Journal of American College of Nutrition* 12 (4), August 1993: 390–99.

'Dietary Fat Intake and Breast Cancer' J. M. Martin Moreno, W. C. Willet, L. Gorgojo, J. R. Benegas, P. Maisoneuve, P. Boyle (Department of Epidemiology and Biostatics, Escuala Nacional de Sanidad, Spain), *International Journal of Cancer*, September 15, 1994: 774–80.

'Diet, Body Build, and Breast Cancer' David J. Hunter and Walter C. Willet (Departments of Epidemiology and Nutrition, Harvard School of Public Health and Channing Laboratory, Department of Medicine, Harvard Medical School, and Brigham and Women's Hospital), *Annual Review of Nutrition* 14, 1994: 393–418.

'Diet and Breast Cancer Risk: Results from a population-based case-controlled study in Sweden' Lars Holmberg, Eva M. Ohlander, Tim Byers, Matthew Zack, Alicia Wolk, Reinhold Bergstrom, Leif Bergkrist, *Arch. Intern. Med* 154, August 22, 1994.

The Directory of Cancer Specialists (The National Cancer Alliance; see Directory for address).

The Directory of Cancer Support and Self Help (CancerLink; see Directory for address).

'Eating fat or Being Fat and Risk of cardiovascular Disease and Cancer Among Women' L. H. Kuller (Department of Epidemiology, Graduate School of Public Health, University of Pittsburgh), *Annual of Epidemiology* 4 (2), March 1994: 119–27.

'Epidemiology of Breast Cancer in Japan' Suketami Tominaga and Tetsua Kuroishi, *Cancer Letters* 90 (1), 23 March 1995: 75–79. Abstract from *Nutrition Research Newsletter*, March 1995, published by Lyda Associates Inc.

A Guide to Breast Cancer in Wales (Tenovus; see Directory for address).

Health of the Nation Report (Department of Health, 1993).

The Holistic Approach to Cancer I. Pearce (C. W. Daniel, 1995).

An Introduction to Psycho-Oncology Patrice Guex (Routledge, 1994).

'Lifetime Alcohol Consumption and Risk of Breast Cancer' Jo L. Freudenheim, James R. Marshall, Saxon Graham *et al.*, *Nutrition and Cancer* 12 (1), 1995: 1–11.

Liz Earle's Lifestyle Guide Liz Earle (Boxtree, 1996).

Macmillan Directory of Breast Cancer Services in the UK (Cancer Relief Macmillan Fund; see Directory for address).

Massage for People with Cancer Patricia McNamara (available from The Cancer Support Centre Wandsworth; see Directory for address).

Menopause & HRT Heather Kirby (Cassell, 1994).

Mixed Messages: Our Breasts in Our Lives Bridgid McConville (Penguin, 1994).

Useful Information

A More Difficult Exercise Diana Moran (Bloomsbury, 1990).

Natural Healing for Women Susan Curtis and Romy Fraser (Pandora, 1991).

Nutrition and Cancer Sandra Goodman (The Green Library, 1995).

'Partial and Complete Regression of Breast Cancer in Patients in Relation to Dosage of Co-enzyme Q10' K. Lockwood, S. Moesgaard, K. Folkers (Pharma Nord, Vejie, Denmark and the Institute for Biomedical Research, University of Texas), *Biochemical and Biophysical Research Communications*, March 30 1994.

Patient No More: The politics of breast cancer Sharon Batt (Scarlet Press, 1995).

'Pesticides Safety Directorate' Ministry of Agriculture, Fisheries and Food, August 1995.

'Pharma Retinol, B-Carotene, and Vitamin E Levels in Relation to the Future Risk of Breast Cancer' N. J. Wald, J. Boreham, J. L. Hayward, R. D. Bulbrook, *British Journal of Cancer* 49, 1984: 321–24.

Preventing Breast Cancer: The politics of an epidemic Dr Cathy Read (Pandora, 1995).

'Serum Vitamins A and E, B-Carotene, and Selenium in Patients with Breast Cancer' Tapan K. Basu, Gerry B. Hill, Ehtesham Abdi, Norman Temple, *The Journal of The American College of Nutrition* 8 (6), 1989: 524–28.

Tamoxifen and Breast Cancer: What everyone should know about the treatment of breast cancer Michael W. de Gregorio and Valerie J. Wiebe (Yale University Press, 1994).

Ultimate Sex Guide Anne Hooper (Dorling Kindersley, 1992).

Well Woman Handbook Denise Winn (Vermilion, 1995).

Well Woman's Self Help Directory Nikki Bradford (Macmillan, 1993).

The Women's Guide to Homoeopathy – the natural way for a healthier life Dr Andrew Lockie & Dr Nicola Geddes (Hamish Hamilton, 1992).

Your Breasts: What every woman needs to know – now Brian H. Butler (T.A.S.K. Books, available from 39 Browns Road, Surbiton, Surrey KT5 8ST).

Contributors

Linda Benn is Head of Cancer Counselling Services at BACUP. 'My interest in cancer, and breast cancer in particular, started long before coming to BACUP when I facilitated a support group for women with cancer. At BACUP both Claire [Crombie] and I work individually with women with breast cancer; they find themselves surprisingly enriched during counselling, and the enrichment continues to be a two-way process.'

Lorraine Butler is assistant editor at *Marie Claire*. 'Two years ago I initiated a campaign at *Today* newspaper to raise money for research. I interviewed Dee Stancombe, a 33-year-old mum who had breast cancer. She died during our campaign; her death made me extremely committed to this cause. *Marie Claire* is also committed to raising funds for research.'

Karena Callen is health & beauty director of British *Cosmopolitan*. She has written *Elle Vitality: A Guide to Health and Beauty* (Ebury), *Dolphins and Their Power to Heal* (Bloomsbury), and *Cosmopolitan's One-to-One Massage* (Ebury). 'Four years ago my friend Karen Hawley died of breast cancer – she was only 33. Since her death I have been committed to raising the awareness of breast cancer in this country, particularly among young women. I would like to dedicate my chapter to the memory of Karen, and to her daughter Catherine.'

Rita Carter is a journalist specializing in health and medicine. She edits the health pages for *She* magazine, and contributes regularly to many newspapers and other magazines, including *Top Sante*, *YOU* (*Mail on Sunday*), *Essentials* and *The Telegraph Magazine*. She also contributes to Radio 4's *Medicine Now*.

Clare Crombie is a BACUP counsellor with a background in education and music.

Susan Curtis has worked with natural remedies since 1979. She trained as a homoeopath, and has since studied and used other forms of natural healing, including herbs, essential oils and flower remedies. Susan practised professionally at a clinic of natural medicine in London, but recently she has committed herself to helping people to treat themselves using natural remedies. She is co-author of *Natural Healing for Women* (Pandora); her latest book is *Neal's Yard Remedies Guide to Essential Oils* (Aurum 1996).

Liz Earle is the bestselling author of more than thirty health and beauty books, and is also known for her regular fashion and lifestyle reports on GMTV. A founder of the Guild of Health Writers, Liz respects the best of both complementary and conventional medicine.

Deborah Fenlon B.Sc. is a clinical nurse specializing in breast care. She has been working at the Royal Marsden NHS Trust for 12 years and caring for women with breast cancer since 1985. As a breast care nurse she has been supporting women through the process of diagnosis and treatment, including the fitting of prostheses, where necessary.

Caryn Franklin was formerly fashion editor and co-editor of *i-D Magazine*. She began working for cable TV in the 1980s and then contributed to a plethora of youth style programmes like *Network 7*, *Tube* and *South of Watford*. She has presented *The Clothes Show* for the last nine years, writing and co-directing various features, including a ten-minute special on eating disorders and fashion imagery, and recently directed and presented a Children in Crisis appeal from Bosnia. Caryn teaches at Central St Martin's and The Surrey Institute, and is external assessor at London College of Fashion. She has directed the campaign video for Fashion Targets Breast Cancer.

Georgina Goodman is a TV and print journalist, as well as a contributing editor to *Elle* magazine. Following the death from breast cancer of a close family member, she has been a keen supporter of breast cancer causes. 'It has been an education and a privilege to work with Caryn, the journalists and all of the medical experts who have contributed to this book. I hope it will be a useful tool in the ongoing campaign to further women's understanding and awareness of breast health.'

Dr Janet Hardy originally trained in medical oncology in New Zealand. She was appointed Head of the Department of Palliative Medicine at the Royal Marsden Hospital NHS Trust in 1991. Her main reason for contributing to this book is her belief that the death of so many women from breast cancer each year cannot be ignored. While it is crucially important to find a cure for this disease, the care and treatment of those patients with incurable breast cancer is also paramount.

Anne Hooper is the author of the bestselling *Ultimate Sex Guide* (Dorling Kindersley), recently released on CD ROM. She is the author of thirteen other books, including *The Body Electric* (Pandora). Anne was the presenter of the former LBC Radio's Counselling Programme for eight years, is presently the Teletext counsellor, and is an accredited sexual and marital therapist, in practice for twenty years. Her latest book is *Anne Hooper's Ultimate Sexual Touch* (Dorling Kindersley).

Deborah Hutton is a contributing editor to *Vogue* magazine, and has been their leading health writer for the last sixteen years; she is also a regular contributor to the health pages of the major national newspapers. As well as having three children and expecting her fourth, she has written three books, the most recent being *Vogue Futures*. Deborah has been a supporter of BREAKTHROUGH Breast Cancer since its beginnings. 'I think BREAKTHROUGH is a dynamic charity perfectly positioned to be the focused force for the change that is so desperately needed.'

Dr Janine L. Mansi has been a Consultant Medical Oncologist at St George's Hospital in London since 1991. During her training she was involved in research into breast cancer at St George's and The Royal Marsden; this particular speciality now forms the largest part of her clinical practice.

Anna Maslin trained as a nurse in 1978, and has been involved in cancer care since 1981; she is currently Breast Group Manager at the Royal Marsden Hospital NHS Trust. She completed a first degree in theology, an MSc in advanced clinical practice and is currently undertaking a part-time Ph.D., looking at patient choice and shared decision-making for women with breast cancer.

Useful Information

Sasha Miller was a writer and editor at the *Sunday Times Magazine* for five years before becoming features editor at *Elle*. She says of Nancy Roberts, 'She is a very inspiring woman and it was a great privilege to meet her. I admire anyone whose reaction to a problem as serious and frightening as breast cancer is to get out there and demand that something positive be done about it.'

Vivienne Parry is a scientist by training but an enthusiast by nature. She is best known as a presenter of BBC TV's popular science show *Tomorrow's World*, but also writes for a wide range of magazines and newspapers. When she arrived at the BBC she was asked to nominate the subject for her first film for *Tomorrow's World*. 'Breast cancer was top of my list – it's not just of immediate concern to everyone, but the subject of some breathtaking new science.'

Nicki Pope was medical correspondent for *Today* newspaper. She now works for the *Daily Express*. 'I'm contributing to this book because my mother, aunt and grandmother have suffered breast cancer.'

Dr Cathy Read is a medical doctor, journalist and author of *Preventing Breast Cancer: the politics of an epidemic* (Pandora), in which she explores the links between lifestyle, environment and breast cancer. She concludes that society could be doing a lot more to protect our children from this devastating but preventable disease.

Dr Ann Robinson works as a GP in north London, and is also writing a book on women's health. 'As a GP, I see a lot of women who are worried about breast lumps or other breast symptoms such as breast pain. I am very interested in promoting breast awareness among all women, identifying those at increased risk of breast cancer so they can be entered in screening programs, and ensuring that my patients who are diagnosed as having breast cancer are offered sympathetic and properly co-ordinated care at a specialist centre.'

Dr Christobel Saunders MB, BS, FRCS is a breast surgeon who originally trained at the Royal Marsden and now lectures at the Breast Unit at Guy's and St Thomas's Hospitals. Her main interests include hormonal aspects of breast cancer, quality of life for the cancer patient and reconstructive breast surgery.

Anna-Marie Solowij has been writing about health and beauty for eight years. She started her career as assistant health and beauty editor at *Marie Claire*, and is currently health and beauty director at *Elle*.

Val Speechley has worked in cancer care for over twenty years. She remained in clinical practice, primarily in chemotherapy and I.V. therapy until seven years ago, when she moved to become the Patient Information Officer at the Royal Marsden Hospital NHS Trust. She is responsible for providing a comprehensive patient information and education service. With Maxine Rosenfield from CancerLink, Val wrote *Cancer Information at Your Fingertips*, which has been recently updated and is recommended by the Cancer Research Campaign.

Sarah Stacey is an award-winning journalist and television researcher/producer, specializing in health. She is currently health editor of *YOU Magazine* (*The Mail on Sunday*) and is Chair of the Guild of Health Writers. Sarah is a regular contributor to the *Daily Telegraph*, the *Evening Standard* and *Good Housekeeping*, and has also written for the *Sunday Times*, *Financial Times*, *Sunday Telegraph*, *Marie Claire Health & Beauty*, *Options*, *She*, *Tatler*, *BBC Wildlife*, *Focus* and *Business Traveller*, amongst others. She is also a director of Paladin Pictures.

Dr Miriam Stoppard is both a respected medical authority and a bestselling author. She has written on the subjects of women's health, pregnancy and baby and child care with a practical, sympathetic approach. Her constant campaigning for greater awareness of women's health issues has brought her further into the public eye, in the form of television appearances and radio interviews. Her books include *Everygirl's Lifeguide*, *Everywoman's Medical Handbook*, *The First Weeks of Life*, *50 Plus Lifeguide*, *The New Baby Care Book*, *The Magic of Sex*, *Woman's Body*, *Conception, Pregnancy and Birth*, *Menopause* and *Complete Baby and Child Care* (all Dorling Kindersley). Dr Stoppard's *Breast Book* (1996) is the first complete illustrated guide to breast care.

Index

Index